THE
EVERYTHING®
GUIDE TO
HERBAL REMEDIES

Dear Reader,

As a devotee of herbal medicine and a self-proclaimed amateur herbalist, I was delighted to take on the task of writing this book. At last, I'd have a chance to talk about the remedies that had been a staple in my medicine cabinet for so many years. Finally, the rest of the world could know the secrets of herbalism.

But as a professional writer and journalist, I approached the subject with a decidedly different attitude: What are these things, really? Who's using them, and why? Do they work? Are they safe? And can the average Joe or Jane find them in the average herb shop or health food store?

I'm happy to report that I've achieved both goals: to get the word out about the many benefits of using herbs, and to explain the traditional uses, supporting research and other evidence, safety concerns, modern uses, and availability of each. I hope you'll agree.

Martha Schindler Connors

Welcome to the EVERYTHING® Series!

These handy, accessible books give you all you need to tackle a difficult project, gain a new hobby, comprehend a fascinating topic, prepare for an exam, or even brush up on something you learned back in school but have since forgotten.

You can choose to read an *Everything*® book from cover to cover or just pick out the information you want from our four useful boxes: e-questions, e-facts, e-alerts, and e-ssentials.

We give you everything you need to know on the subject, but throw in a lot of fun stuff along the way, too.

We now have more than 400 *Everything*® books in print, spanning such wide-ranging categories as weddings, pregnancy, cooking, music instruction, foreign language, crafts, pets, New Age, and so much more. When you're done reading them all, you can finally say you know *Everything*®!

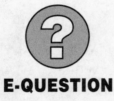

E-QUESTION
Answers to
common questions

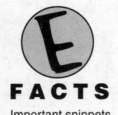

FACTS
Important snippets
of information

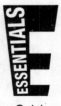

ALERTS!
Urgent
warnings

ESSENTIALS
Quick
handy tips

PUBLISHER Karen Cooper

DIRECTOR OF ACQUISITIONS AND INNOVATION Paula Munier

MANAGING EDITOR, EVERYTHING SERIES Lisa Laing

COPY CHIEF Casey Ebert

ACQUISITIONS EDITOR Lisa Laing

SENIOR DEVELOPMENT EDITOR Brett Palana-Shanahan

EDITORIAL ASSISTANT Hillary Thompson

Visit the entire Everything® series at *www.everything.com*

THE
EVERYTHING®
GUIDE TO HERBAL REMEDIES

An easy-to-use reference for natural health care

Martha Schindler Connors with Larry Altshuler, MD

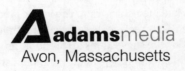

Adamsmedia
Avon, Massachusetts

This book is dedicated to my husband, Don, who is my inspiration in all things (including herbs).

An Everything® Series Book.
Everything® and everything.com® are registered trademarks of F+W Media, Inc.

Published by Adams Media, a division of F+W Media, Inc.
57 Littlefield Street, Avon, MA 02322 U.S.A.
www.adamsmedia.com

ISBN 10: 1-59869-988-1
ISBN 13: 978-1-59869-988-3

Printed in the United States of America.

J   I   H   G   F   E   D   C   B   A

Library of Congress Cataloging-in-Publication Data
is available from the publisher.

This publication is designed to provide accurate and authoritative information with regard to the subject matter covered. It is sold with the understanding that the publisher is not engaged in rendering legal, accounting, or other professional advice. If legal advice or other expert assistance is required, the services of a competent professional person should be sought.

—From a *Declaration of Principles* jointly adopted by a Committee of the American Bar Association and a Committee of Publishers and Associations

Many of the designations used by manufacturers and sellers to distinguish their products are claimed as trademarks. Where those designations appear in this book and Adams Media was aware of a trademark claim, the designations have been printed with initial capital letters.

This book is available at quantity discounts for bulk purchases.
For information, please call 1-800-289-0963.

The Everything® Guide to Herbal Remedies is intended as a reference volume only, not as a medical manual. In light of the complex, individual, and specific nature of health problems, this book is not intended to replace professional medical advice. The ideas, procedures, and suggestions in this book are intended to supplement, not replace, the advice of a trained medical professional. Consult your physician before adopting the suggestions in this book, as well as about any condition that may require diagnosis or medical attention. The author and publisher disclaim any liability arising directly or indirectly from the use of this book.

Contents

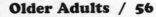

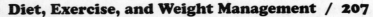

Acknowledgments

Many thanks to Rosemary Gladstar and the other herbalists, researchers, doctors, and others who helped me pull this book together.

Top Ten Ways to Ease Herbs into Your Health Care Routine

1. Add antioxidant foods (like tomatoes and spinach) and herbs and spices (like turmeric and rosemary) to your pantry.

2. Toss the hydrogen peroxide and get some tea tree oil instead.

3. Visit an herb shop and check out the bulk herb section. Open each jar, give it a good sniff, and go home with at least one bag of dried plant matter (see Chapter 19 for tips on what to do with it).

4. Ease yourself to sleep with a massage using lavender essential oil (you might need a partner for this one).

5. Add some digestion-friendly flaxseeds to your oatmeal.

6. Take a walk (and some lemon balm) the next time you're feeling stressed.

7. Give your hair color a boost with a rinse made with chamomile or black tea.

8. Substitute a cup of mate or rooibos tea for your usual morning coffee.

9. Replace your bath bubbles with a few drops of rose essential oil.

10. Skip the colds this winter with astragalus.

Introduction

▶ HERBAL MEDICINE WAS, until fairly recently, the only kind of medicine. Since human beings started recording their history—and probably long before that—nearly every imaginable remedy came from plants.

Yet somewhere along the line, medicine took a turn away from herbalism, and the two have been running on parallel tracks ever since. While "conventional" once was synonymous with "herbal," it gradually came to mean something completely different.

As doctors and scientists began to make the connection between chemistry and disease, plants were scrutinized and synthesized and eventually replaced by pharmaceuticals, which could deliver swifter and more powerful results. Herbal remedies fell by the wayside, regarded by most people as quaint and folksy, something left to the fringe of modern medicine.

Yet as we developed more and more powerful weapons against disease—things like chemotherapy and radiation, steroidal painkillers and antibiotics—many people began searching for something else. What if you didn't need the big guns of conventional medicine? What if you didn't have cancer or cardiovascular disease and just wanted to avoid getting the flu? Or to stave off problems like cancer and heart disease before they even began?

Enter herbs—again. Unlike conventional drugs and treatments, herbs can treat chronic and acute conditions, but they're also effective tools for maintaining overall health. Many herbs boost the immune system; others naturally regulate hormone levels or lower blood sugar and cholesterol levels.

The traditions of herbal medicine are grounded in a basic belief: that the body is naturally healthy and balanced, and that it can remain that way—or be eased back into its balanced position—through the judicious use of remedies like herbs. Like human beings, plants are natural and complete organisms that have adapted and survived over the millennia by developing natural defenses against their enemies. Herbal medicine harnesses those properties to create remedies that can help you, too.

The last several years have seen a resurgence of herbal medicine, as millions of people search for gentle, natural alternatives to conventional medicine. Recently, the World Health Organization (WHO) estimated that 65 percent of people worldwide rely on herbal medicines for some aspect of their primary health care. In Germany, roughly 600 to 700 plant-based medicines are available and are prescribed by approximately 70 percent of German physicians. Herbal remedies are recognized as legitimate forms of medicine in most countries today.

In the United States, herbalism is classified as a type of complementary and alternative medicine, or CAM, a group of practices that can be used as adjuncts to conventional medical care. The National Institutes of Health (NIH) and the National Center for Complementary and Alternative Medicine (NCCAM) now support clinical trials on specific herbs. Millions of Americans—more than a third of all adults—are using herbs and other types of CAM. NCCAM reports that roughly one-fifth of U.S. adults incorporate herbs and other natural agents into their health care routines. Of the most commonly used products, nine out of ten were herbs (the only nonherb was fish oil).

Yet herbs and herbal remedies are the subject of much debate, as herbal practitioners, medical doctors, scientists, and politicians wrestle with some important questions: How should herbs be treated? Are they drugs, comparable to prescription and nonprescription pharmaceuticals? Or are they dietary supplements, a kind of glorified food product more like vitamins and minerals? Should herbs be completely deconstructed, with each individual compound identified and quantified? Because they contain so many chemicals, each with a specific action that can trigger complex physiological responses—and potentially create side effects or problems when combined with conventional drugs—should herbal products carry warning labels? Officially, herbs are viewed and monitored as supplements, without the requirement for such tight scrutiny or labeling, but the case is far from closed.

Most experts agree that herbs possess unique yet tangible benefits, and that they can be used to complement conventional treatments and enhance overall health. Using herbs safely and effectively means understanding their powers—and limitations—and treating them like the medicines they are.

CHAPTER 1

What Is Herbal Medicine?

Herbal medicine, also called *botanical medicine* or *phytomedicine*, is the practice of using one or more parts of a plant—its seeds, berries, roots, leaves, bark, or flowers—to relieve physical and psychological problems, prevent disease, or just improve overall health and vitality. Although many modern drugs were originally developed from plants, they are based on isolated chemicals, while plants comprise myriad active components, which work together to create their medicinal actions. Herbs have a long history of use and, when used properly, are safe and powerful medicines.

The History of Herbal Healing

Long before doctors in lab coats started writing prescriptions—in fact, even before human beings started writing at all—herbs were being used as medicine. Herbal medicine has prehistoric origins, and it continues today in virtually every culture in the world.

Herbal medicine dates back thousands of years, although no one is exactly sure when the first human used an herb to treat a health woe. In the American Southwest, for example, researchers have found human genetic material on hunks (called *quids*) of the herb yucca, which were chewed and spit out like a kind of ancient chewing gum. The quids are between 800 and 2,400 years old.

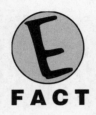

The World Health Organization reports that roughly 25 percent of all modern medicines are made from plants that came straight out of traditional medicine. For example, two South American species, the chinchona tree (*Chinchona officinalis*) and the coca plant (*Erythroxylum coca*), have given us the antimalaria drug quinine and several types of anesthetics.

In Europe, researchers discovered what looks to be herbal remedies on the body of the infamous "Ice Man," the 3,000-year-old mummy discovered in the early 1990s in the Italian Alps. Researchers found walnut-sized lumps of birch fungus, which has laxative and antibiotic properties, on his body. An autopsy revealed that the man had been suffering from an infestation of parasitic whipworms, leading the experts to guess that he had most likely been treating them with measured doses of the medicine.

As civilizations rose up around the world, so did herbal medicine. And although some of the ancients' remedies have fallen by the wayside, most are still popular.

The Egyptian priest and physician Imhotep, who lived around 2600 B.C. and is often credited with the earliest medical writings, described the diagnoses and treatments—many of them herbal—of more than 200 diseases.

In China, the emperor Shen Nung, in 2735 B.C., wrote what is generally believed to be the earliest treatise on herbs, discussing hundreds of medicinal plants that are still in use. And in India, a manuscript from around 2000 B.C. mentions the herbs cinnamon, ginger, and sandalwood as ingredients in several medical preparations.

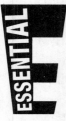

To avoid confusion (and language barriers), an herb is usually identified by its common name as well as its scientific (botanical) name, which comprises the Latin words for the plant's genus and species. That way, if you're looking for chamomile, you'll know if you're getting the popular German or Hungarian variety (*Matricaria recutita*) or the less common Roman or English variety (*Chamaemelum nobile*).

Principles and Traditions

No matter where in the world it originated, any school of traditional herbal medicine is based on a simple concept: that herbal remedies can be used to create—or re-create—a state of health within the body. Herbal healers categorize diseases according to a specific set of symptoms, then use their remedies to restore the patient to the state he was in before the disease struck.

A "Humor"ous Approach

Western herbalism evolved from the Greeks, who in turn were strongly influenced by Egyptian and Middle Eastern civilizations. The Greek system uses a system of "*humors*," which are tied to four dynamic elements (air, earth, water, and fire). The Greeks believed that diseases were caused by an imbalance of these humors. The humors were part of an individual's nature and weren't necessarily good or bad. But if they got out of balance, illness would ensue.

The theory of the humors is similar to the basic beliefs of Traditional Chinese Medicine (TCM) and Ayurvedic medicine, which originated in India at roughly the same time. In Ayurveda, for example, there are three *doshas*, or body types, which correspond to the natural world and also reflect an individual's innate nature.

Actions Speak Louder

Traditional herbal medicine is also organized around each herb's physiological actions—what it does in the body. (Not surprisingly, modern herbalists do the same thing.) For example, the Greeks categorized their herbs as warming, drying, cooling, binding, and relaxing. The Chinese have classifications like purging, lubricating, stimulating, clearing, and calming. Not too far from our modern-day classifications, which you'll see as you walk down the aisle of any drug store: expectorants, laxatives, sedatives, stimulants, and so on.

And while some consumers might scoff at some traditional terminology, modern research shows that, for the most part, the ancients had it right. In fact, of the 100-plus known medicinal plant compounds used today, roughly 80 percent are used for purposes that are identical or very close to their traditional use.

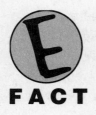

FACT

One of the most powerful chemotherapy agents existing today comes from the Pacific yew (*Taxus brevifolia*). Yew trees were routinely discarded in logging enterprises until 1967, when somebody discovered a compound called *taxol* that could inhibit the division of cancerous cells. Today, taxol is used to treat breast, ovarian, and lung cancer.

The Chemistry of Plants

Although people have been using herbs for centuries, we don't know a whole lot about the pharmacology, or chemical makeup, of many of them. Unlike pharmaceuticals—drugs created in a lab from a precise chemical recipe—herbs are often chemical mysteries.

Unraveling the Mysteries

In recent years, scientists have been deconstructing herbs to determine the chemical compounds—called *phytochemicals*—behind their actions.

For example, researchers have determined that garlic (*Allium sativum*) owes much of its antibacterial and cholesterol-lowering action to a phytochemical called allicin. Ginger (*Zingiber officinale*) apparently gets its stomach-settling powers from two chemicals, 6-gingerol and gingerdione. And cayenne peppers (*Capsicum annuum, C. frutescens*) contain capsaicin, which dulls pain and produces a warming sensation.

Primary and Secondary

In most cases, the compounds that are so helpful to humans are actually secondary to the plant's survival. The most important things, at least as far as the plant is concerned, are the *primary constituents*, which are used in the plant's primary metabolic processes (like photosynthesis) and include things like sugars and chlorophyll.

Secondary constituents are things that the plant developed over the course of its evolution to defend itself against animals, insects, disease, or environmental stresses such as changes in temperature or water levels. Quite often these compounds—which include vitamins, minerals, essential oils, and phytochemicals—are key to both the plant's viability and its bioactivity (the effect it has on another living organism or tissue).

ESSENTIAL

According to the latest estimates, there are 122 scientifically identified plant compounds being used as drugs throughout the world, which are drawn from just 94 plant species. With several thousand known medicinal plants now in use, scientists still have quite a few more chemicals to name.

Luckily, the chemicals that make a plant unappealing to microbes can serve as antimicrobial agents in humans, too. And the neurotoxic chemicals that a plant uses to defend itself against foraging deer can work as sedatives, muscle relaxants, or anesthetics in people.

Most of the secondary constituents in plants can be lumped into three categories: terpenoids, alkaloids, and polyphenols.

Terpenoids

Many terpenoids are either toxic or just unappetizing to grazing animals; others make a plant more appealing to pollinating insects. Feverfew (*Tanacetum parthenium*) and chamomile (*Matricaria recutita*) contain medicinal terpenoids.

Alkaloids

Alkaloids can have potent medicinal activity. Examples are nitrogen, caffeine, quinine, morphine, and nicotine. The Chinese herb ma huang (*Ephedra sinica*) contains the alkaloid ephedrine. Cocaine is found in the leaves of the coca shrub (*Erythroxylum coca*).

Polyphenols

Polyphenols include tannins and flavonoids. Tannins are astringent chemicals (once used to tan animal hides) found in the seeds and stems of grapes (*Vitis vinifera*), the leaves and bark of trees or shrubs like witch hazel (*Hamamelis virginiana*), and tea leaves (*Camellia sinensis*). Flavonoids are a broad class of compounds that act as *antioxidants* (agents that counteract the process of oxidation, which can damage cells and trigger disease). They are found in ginkgo (*Ginkgo biloba*), hawthorn (*Crataegus monogyna, C. oxyacantha*), and milk thistle (*Silybum marianum*), among others. Isoflavones are one type of flavonoid that act as *phytoestrogens* (plant compounds that mimic the effects of estrogen in the body). Isoflavones are found in soybeans (*Glycine max*).

The Sum Versus the Whole

But while scientists have identified the active constituents in many herbs, many more remain a mystery, in part because the chemicals in the plant appear to work synergistically instead of individually.

That means that, in most cases, we don't know which ingredient in a plant is causing a therapeutic effect, or if that ingredient is acting alone or in combination with other ingredients. Moreover, because it's a natural thing, an herb's biochemical composition is inherently variable and can change from year to year or crop to crop.

The Evolution of Herbal Medicine

As early civilizations developed, they slowly left behind the hunting-and-gathering routine in favor of cultivation, building settlements, and developing a more cohesive social structure. In virtually every part of the world, herbs were part of the arsenal of healers, who combined spiritual and religious elements in their medicine.

ALERT!

Before test tubes and research labs, herbalists around the world used a decidedly nonscientific method called "the doctrine of signatures," which held that plants (or plant parts) that looked like a human body part would benefit that part. Thus, medieval healers recommended the phallus-shaped mandrake (*Mandragora officinarum*) root for impotence and the brainy-looking walnut (*Juglans regia*) for mental disorders.

As people began to grow and gather herbs, they learned, through experience, trial-and-error, and plain old luck, which plants could be useful and which ought to be avoided.

To help them understand the complexities of their world, primitive people came up with a pantheon of gods, spirits, and supernatural forces, many of which were directly tied to the natural world. In time, people around the world began to realize that sickness and disease (or health and vitality, for that matter) were created by natural and not supernatural processes. At that point, the healing profession split into separate factions, with the physician on one side and the priest on the other.

In the early nineteenth century, scientists began extracting and modifying the active ingredients from plants and transforming those ingredients into synthetic drugs. Gradually, medicine—and popular tastes—shifted from herbals to pharmaceuticals.

In 1820, the U.S. Pharmacopeia (USP) published its first standards compendium, then consisting of only natural medicines. But things were changing, and in the United States and many other Western countries, herbal medicine was quickly moving from its place as the primary health care system to a type of supplemental care.

Many countries, including India and Germany, now consider many herbs to be medicines (and therefore regulate them as drugs). According to the latest report from the World Health Organization (WHO), ninety-two countries have an official registration system for herbal medicines, and seventeen of them have more than 1,000 herbal medicines registered.

ESSENTIAL

In the United States, herbs have been regulated by the Food and Drug Administration (FDA) and its predecessor agencies for the past 100 years. In 1994, the government passed the Dietary Supplement Health and Education Act (DSHEA), which classified nearly all herbal products as dietary supplements—to be handled like foods, not medicines.

How Herbs Can Complement Conventional Medicine

Until recently, herbal medicine was practiced outside of conventional medicine, the system of pharmaceuticals and surgery that most Americans think of when they think of health care. But these days, herbalism is going mainstream, as more and more people catch on to its benefits—and more and more studies show the power of plants in treating and preventing disease. The various schools of complementary and alternative treatments (including herbal medicine) are known collectively as CAM. Combining CAM with conventional medicine is known as integrative medicine.

Working Together

Although you should always consult a medical professional in the case of a serious injury or chronic disease, you can use herbs to treat many minor health problems and to maintain your overall health. And with your doctor's approval, you also can add herbs to many conventional medical treatments. In many cases, you don't need the firepower that pharmaceutical drugs provide; the gentler properties of herbs will serve you much better.

Indeed, one of the biggest selling points for many MDs is the disease-preventing power that many herbs have. Research continues to show that various preventive measures—getting enough exercise, eating healthy foods, etc.—can stave off many diseases, and herbs with nutritional value fit the bill nicely. Consider the case of antioxidants, a class of plant chemicals that prevent cell damage caused by reactive molecules known as free radicals. Research shows certain micronutrients—most notably vitamins C and E and the mineral selenium—have high antioxidant levels. But many medicinal and culinary herbs are also antioxidant powerhouses. Some of the biggest include tea (*Camellia sinensis*), elderberry (*Sambucus nigra*), rosemary (*Rosmarinus officinalis*), and turmeric (*Curcuma longa*).

Common Ground

Herbs also can work as complementary or adjunct therapies, enhancing the effects of conventional drugs and/or treatments and offsetting any side effects they might produce.

For example, ginger (*Zingiber officinale*) can relieve post-operative and chemotherapy-induced nausea.

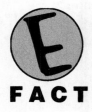

FACT

Tea (*Camellia sinensis*) is the world's second most popular beverage (behind water). It comes in three varieties: green, which is unfermented, oolong, which is partially fermented, and black, which is completely fermented. All are good for you, but green tea seems to have the highest levels of polyphenols, the phytochemicals credited with many of tea's benefits.

In other cases, herbs can accentuate the benefits of conventional treatments. For example, cancer patients who take cordyceps mushrooms (*Cordyceps sinensis*) after chemotherapy treatments seem to get a boost in cellular immunity. And a new study shows that combining chemotherapy with the Chinese herb astragalus (*Astragalus membranaceus*) works better than chemotherapy alone at stimulating the patient's immune system. Other studies have shown that the turkey tail, or coriolus, mushroom (*Trametes versicolor*,

Coriolus versicolor) can significantly prolong cancer survival when taken in conjunction with chemotherapy or radiation treatment.

Other Healing (Herbal) Modalities

Many health care professionals, including naturopathic physicians, chiropractors, and practitioners of Traditional Chinese Medicine (TCM) and Ayurveda (the ancient system of health care of India), use herbs and herbal formulations. Herbs also play a part in other types of natural health care, including aromatherapy and homeopathy.

Aromatherapy

Aromatherapy is the practice of using aromatic plants to treat various conditions and maintain overall health. It dates back to the ancient Egyptians, Greeks, and Romans, who used fragrant plant oils in healing baths and therapeutic massage.

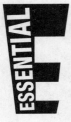

Legend has it that modern "aromatherapy" was born in the 1920s, when a French chemist inadvertently discovered the power of plant oils when he burned his hand and plunged it into the nearest cool liquid he could find: a vat of lavender oil. The pain was relieved and the burn healed remarkably well, with no inflammation, blistering, or scarring.

Modern aromatherapy uses *essential oils*, which are volatile liquids distilled in a way that selects miniscule molecules and leaves behind heavier plant waxes, oils, and other materials. Thus, essential oils are incredibly potent and deliver what the experts consider to be the "essential" parts of the plant: its phytochemicals and its scent.

Today, aromatherapy is practiced by aerial diffusion, direct inhalation, and topical application (via massage). Experts theorize that it works in two ways. The first is through aroma, which moves through the olfactory system to stimulate limbic (emotional) centers of the brain. The other is through a direct pharmacological effect: The oils' beneficial compounds are delivered via the skin or mucous membranes.

Homeopathy

Homeopathy is a school of natural medicine developed in eighteenth-century Germany and based on a simple theory, called "the law of similars," which holds that a substance that produces symptoms in a healthy person will cure a sick person showing the same symptoms (the word *homeopathy* comes from two Greek words: *homoios*, meaning "similar," and *pathos*, meaning "sickness"). In shorthand: "Like cures like."

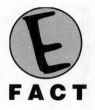

FACT

The "like cures like" theory of homeopathy is not as far-out as it might seem. It's actually rooted in ancient Greek tradition, where it was called *similia similibus curentur,* or the "similia principle." Centuries before homeopathy was developed, Hippocrates had found that he could treat recurrent vomiting with an emetic herb (one that would ordinarily be used to induce vomiting).

The other basic tenet of homeopathy is the law of potentization, which holds that the lower the dose of a medicine, the greater its potency—and effect. Homeopathic remedies are sold according to their potency: The ingredients are diluted, then shaken over and over again (in a process called *succussion*) until there are only miniscule amounts of the original compound (or none at all) remaining.

Many homeopathic remedies are derived from plants, and others use minerals and animal parts.

Flower Essences

Flower essences, also known as flower remedies, were developed in the early twentieth century by British physician and homeopath Edward Bach (pronounced "Batch"), who felt that many, if not all, of the physical problems people face are tied to our emotional state. According to Bach, you could be healthy only after you cast out the negative emotions—fear, worry, animosity, and indecision—that destroy your body's equilibrium.

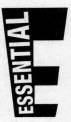

The most famous flower essence product is known as "five-flower remedy" and sold under various names (the most popular of which is Bach's Rescue Remedy). It's a premixed combination of the essences of cherry plum, clematis, impatiens, rock rose, and star of Bethlehem, used to relieve the stress caused by travel, injury, or an upcoming event.

Bach came up with thirty-eight flower remedies, all based on the homeopathic principles of similarity and potency. He chose flowers that reflect the condition that needs attention (the aspen tree, which seems to quake before a storm, gives us the remedy for anxiety and apprehension, while impatiens is prescribed for individuals who are hasty and—you guessed it—impatient).

Healing Foods

Herbs can also be incorporated into the menu, and they deliver their benefits as easily when they're served as a food as when they're taken as medicine. Edible herbs with proven health benefits are called *functional foods*.

Medicinal Mushrooms

Several varieties of edible mushrooms are considered medicinal. In particular, reishi (*Ganoderma lucidum*), shiitake (*Lentinula edodes*), and maitake (*Grifola frondosa*) appear to support immunity, fight infection, and even offer protection against diabetes, heart disease, and cancer. Mushrooms contain carbohydrates called *polysaccharides*, which stimulate the immune system. Some specifically stimulate the "natural killer" cells, which can recognize and attack cancer cells.

Many types of mushrooms are also loaded with antioxidants, and studies show that some varieties have more antioxidant power than brightly colored vegetables like carrots and tomatoes.

Studies suggest that other polysaccharides may help protect bone marrow from the effects of chemotherapy and enhance its ability to fight cancer. Research also shows that mushrooms typically contain large levels of a material called *chitin*, which can lower cholesterol.

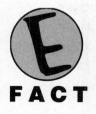

FACT

It's not just the gourmet fungi that have benefits: Inedible mushrooms can pack a real medicinal punch, too. For instance, a recent study found that dried extracts of the cordyceps mushroom (*Cordyceps sinensis*), a mainstay of Chinese medicine, appear to increase aerobic fitness in middle-aged adults.

Soy

Eating soybeans (or soy-based products like tofu and tempeh) has been proven to improve your health in many ways. The *isoflavones* in soy have proven anti-inflammatory, pain-relieving, and cancer-fighting benefits; eating soy has also been linked to a reduction of menopausal symptoms such as hot flashes.

Garlic and Onions

They might wreak havoc on your breath, but these two herbs—actually part of the same genus of plants—can do wonders for your health.

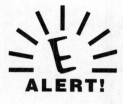

ALERT!

In order to reap the benefits of fresh garlic, you've got to eat it raw, as any cooking dramatically reduces its disease-fighting activity. And don't eat the cloves whole—garlic's active constituent, *allicin*, is created when the enzyme *allinase* is released by chopping or crushing the cloves and exposing them to air for more than ten minutes.

Studies show that both onions (*Allium cepa*) and garlic (*Allium sativum*) contain *sulfur compounds* that can help with diabetes, heart disease, and cancer. In other research, garlic has been shown to prevent artery damage caused by LDL—or "bad"—cholesterol.

Ginger

Ginger (*Zingiber officinale*) is a healthy addition to many dishes, whether you use the root fresh or dried and powdered. Studies show that it can reduce many types of pain and inflammation, including the type associated with rheumatoid and osteoarthritis.

Ginger can also relieve nausea and vomiting from many causes, including seasickness, anesthesia, and pregnancy.

Cocoa

Eating dark chocolate made from *Theobroma cacao* has proven health benefits, including lowering blood pressure, improving cholesterol levels, fighting age-related cognitive decline, preventing blood clots during prolonged travel, and even reducing the risk of certain cancers. And drinking cocoa helps, too. A new study found that older men (aged sixty-five to eighty-four) who consumed the most cocoa had half the risk of dying during the study's fifteen-year span than those who got none.

Why Herbal Medicine Works

Herbalism has a long history of efficacy and safety, and has earned its place in the pantheon of modern medicine. Here's why:

Many herbal remedies have hundreds, if not thousands, of years behind them. And while pharmaceuticals are often tested for short-term safety only, drugs that have been used as folk medicine over millennia have been proven safe and effective over the long term.

Moreover, herbs are generally used for more than one condition, as opposed to drugs, most of which are used for a single purpose.

Of course, there are exceptions to this rule, but generally speaking, herbs are much easier on your body than their pharmaceutical counterparts. Consider the drugs used for depression: Side effects for popular antidepressants like Prozac and Celexa include impaired thinking, sexual problems, insomnia, and headaches. In contrast, herbal remedies like lemon balm (*Melissa officinalis*), rhodiola (*Rhodiola rosea*), and Saint John's wort (*Hypericum perforatum*) fight depression with relatively few unwanted effects.

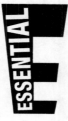

> Traditional and herbal medicine is the main type of health care for most of the planet's population, and the use of complementary and alternative medicine is rising throughout the world. In some countries, up to 80 percent of people consider herbs to be their primary method of staying well.

The basic tenet of herbalism—and all schools of natural medicine—is that it's better to work for optimal health all the time than to wait until disease strikes. For example, herbalists have long recommended herbs like American ginseng (*Panax quinquefolius*) to help stave off the common cold. And a new study shows that consuming dried extracts of the herb reduces both the incidence and the severity of colds.

Additionally, herbs contain many constituents that work together to alleviate specific symptoms—and to address an underlying problem and strengthen the overall functioning of a particular organ or system. And herbs are often used together to foster health.

For example, a multiherb combination containing licorice (*Glycyrrhiza glabra*), chamomile (*Matricaria recutita*), peppermint (*Mentha x piperita*), and lemon balm (*Melissa officinalis*) is used to treat heartburn, nausea, and vomiting—and strengthen the digestive system.

Lastly, it's a rare herb that's used to treat just one body part or system. Most treat several things at once—and new research is backing up that whole-body approach. Consider green tea (*Camellia sinensis*): It's been associated with head-to-toe benefits ranging from reduced cognitive decline, lowered incidence of heart disease and many cancers, and improvements in overall mortality rates. It's used successfully to fight oral bacteria, allergies, bladder infections, and genital warts—and even appears effective against antibiotic-resistant "superbugs." Try to find a drug or therapy in conventional medicine that can make those claims.

CHAPTER 2

Herbs and Their Actions

Herbs are, without question, the first drugs that humans have ever had. And over the centuries, our herbal pharmacy has expanded to include thousands of medicinal plants, each containing a blend of constituents that we're only now beginning to understand. But the real appeal of herbal medicine, of course, is what it can do for you: what diseases it can cure, what complaints it can fix, and how it can make you feel better overall.

Types of Herbs

Herbal remedies are most easily understood when they're grouped according to the jobs they do within the human body. There are hundreds of medicinal herbs out there, and herbalists break them down a few ways:

A *tonic* is an herb that is used to address the health of an entire bodily system. Some tonics also work as *adaptogens* (see below). Tonics can be taken for an extended period of time, like a multivitamin, to keep things running smoothly. They're nontoxic and considered completely safe when used correctly.

Specifics are used to treat a specific symptom—a stomachache, for example. They are taken for a short time only, until the problem is resolved (or until you decide to try a different remedy). Specifics are also generally safe, but they can cause problems if you take too much of them.

In Traditional Chinese Medicine (TCM), tonics are considered "superior" medicines because they can be taken safely and without ill effects for long periods of time. Most other medicinal herbs are considered "ministerial," or "common." They're stronger and work faster, but can be problematic if taken for too long.

Many herbs have more than one action, and some work as tonics in one system and as specifics in another.

Herbs are also classified according to their actions. For example, some trigger a response in the digestive system (they include carminatives and digestives), and others address the nervous system (sedatives and stimulants).

Tonics and Adaptogens

Tonics and adaptogens are a unique type of medicine. They produce what herbalists call a "nonspecific" response, meaning that depending on the organ or system that's being treated, the herb might improve your physical endurance, reproductive and sexual functioning, or resistance to disease.

Tonic Herbs

Tonic herbs are defined as those that address the health of an entire bodily system and alleviate weakness.

In Traditional Chinese Medicine (TCM), tonics are known as superior medicines—the best of the best—and are typically used to strengthen and fortify a system that needs "toning" or "tonifying" (it's failing or just not performing optimally).

There are herbs that have general tonic abilities, meaning they're used to increase your overall energy, or *chi*. Other TCM tonics address specific systems and functions, and some have more than one kind of tonic activity:

- **Astragalus** (*Astragalus membranaceus*) is an immune tonic.
- **Cordyceps** (*Cordyceps sinensis*) is a kidney and adrenal tonic.
- **Eleuthero** (*Eleutherococcus senticosus*) is an immune and chi tonic.
- **Goji-berry** (*Lycium barbarum, L. chinense*) is an immune tonic and blood tonic.
- **Reishi** (*Ganoderma lucidum*) is a heart tonic.

Ayurvedic medicine recognizes a class of herbs known as *rasayanas*, or rejuvenating medicines, that are similar to tonics in that they support the overall functioning of the major systems of the body. The rasayanas include:

- **Amla** (*Emblica officinalis, Phyllanthus emblica*)
- **Gotu kola** (*Centella asiatica*)
- **Tulsi** (*Ocimum tenuiflorum, O. sanctum*)
- **Turmeric** (*Curcuma longa*)

Western herbalism recognizes a group of herbs that work as *nervines*, or nerve tonics, helping to restore balance to the nervous system and emotions and treat problems in the digestive and cardiovascular systems that are caused by anxiety and stress. Nervines include:

- **Chamomile** (*Matricaria recutita*)
- **Hawthorn** (*Crataegus monogyna, C. oxyacantha*)
- **Lemon balm** (*Melissa officinalis*)
- **Passionflower** (*Passiflora incarnata*)
- **Reishi** (*Ganoderma lucidum*)
- **Skullcap** (*Scutellaria lateriflora*)
- **Saint John's wort** (*Hypericum perforatum*)

Adaptogens

An *adaptogen* is something that protects an organism from the ill effects of stress, which can be caused by both physical and psychological agents. In herbal medicine, an adaptogenic herb is one that helps the body deal with stresses—trauma, injury, emotional upset, physical exertion, and so on—without getting sick.

The Stress Response

Stress is defined as the disruption of the body's innate balance, or *homeostasis*, through external agents, and the body's response to it.

In most cases, the stress response is a good thing: It helped our ancestors outrun predators, fight for mates, and survive those cold nights in the cave. But sometimes, stress can be bad. Chronic stress has been linked to a host of diseases and conditions, including premenstrual syndrome (PMS), obesity, insomnia, diarrhea and constipation, anxiety and depression, and suppressed immunity—which can lead to everything from the common cold to cancer.

The Advantage of Adaptogens

Like tonics, adaptogenic plants offer what scientists call "nonspecific" resistance to stress and fatigue, eliminating or reducing the variations in homeostasis that stress produces. They take things a step further, however, by exerting a normalizing effect on an organ or system.

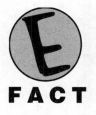

FACT

The term *adaptogen* was coined in Western medicine in the twentieth century, but in the ancient schools of TCM and Ayurveda, the concept has been around for centuries. TCM has chi tonics and Ayurvedic medicine has rasayanas, which have similar properties. Many tonics and rasayanas are also considered adaptogens.

Adaptogens help the body adapt by either increasing or decreasing a particular physiological function. Thus, if something—your adrenal response, for example—needs to be turned on, an adaptogen can do it.

And if that system needs to be turned down, an adaptogen can do that, too.

Here are some of the best—the best-known and best-researched—herbal adaptogens:

- Ashwagandha (*Withania somnifera*)
- Asian ginseng (*Panax ginseng*)
- Cordyceps (*Cordyceps sinensis*)
- Licorice (*Glycyrrhiza glabra*)

- Rhodiola (*Rhodiola rosea*)
- Schisandra (*Schisandra chinensis*)
- Tulsi (*Ocimum tenuiflorum, O. sanctum*)

Analgesics: Natural Pain Relief

An analgesic is a painkiller (the word *analgesia* comes from the Greek words *an*, meaning "without," and *algia*, or "pain").

Herbal analgesics are considered superior to pharmaceutical painkillers such as ibuprofen because they don't carry the same side effects. Herbal pain remedies often work as well as pharmaceuticals, and many are used topically (applied to the skin instead of being ingested), which makes their effects more targeted.

ESSENTIAL

Perhaps the best-known analgesic in the world is morphine, which is derived from the sap of opium poppies (*Papaver somniferum*). First used by the ancient Sumerians, who called poppies "the joy plant," opium was the gold standard in painkillers throughout the world for another 5,000 years.

Here are some of the more popular herbal painkillers:

- Camphor (*Cinnamomum camphora*)
- Cayenne (*Capsicum annuum, C. frutescens*)
- Devil's claw (*Harpagophytum procumbens*)

- Feverfew (*Tanacetum parthenium*)
- Goldenseal (*Hydrastis canadensis*)
- Willow (*Salix alba*)

Fighting Inflammation

An anti-inflammatory agent is anything that reduces inflammation—redness, tenderness, and swelling (or *edema*)—in the tissues. Anti-inflammatories are often effective analgesics as well, since inflammation frequently produces pain along with swelling.

Although it's the source of many health problems, inflammation can actually be a good thing—it's the body's way of protecting itself from injury or infection. Problems start when inflammation gets out of hand or goes on for too long. Chronic inflammation can cause swelling and discomfort that never go away and can damage cartilage, bone, and other tissues.

The first choice in over-the-counter (OTC) pain medicines for most Americans is a *nonsteroidal anti-inflammatory drug*, or NSAID. Most NSAIDs work by inhibiting enzymes (two types of cyclooxygenase enzymes, called *COX-1* and *COX-2*) that produce pain and inflammation.

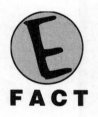

Several herbs, including the African plant devil's claw (*Harpagophytum procumbens*), turmeric (*Curcuma longa*), and phyllanthus (*Phyllanthus amarus*), an Ayurvedic herb also known as bahupatra, have shown drug-like COX-2-inhibiting activity in studies, meaning they could be used as alternative remedies in cases of severe pain as well as everyday aches.

NSAIDs are the most widely used type of pain relief in the United States, and include OTC remedies like ibuprofen (Advil), naproxen (Aleve), and aspirin, and prescription COX-2 inhibitors like celecoxib (Celebrex). NSAIDs can cause a host of problems, including serious kidney, heart, and gastrointestinal problems like ulceration, bleeding, and perforation of the stomach.

In many cases, herbal anti-inflammatories provide the same kind of relief as pharmaceuticals—without the scary side effects. Here are some of the best-known herbal anti-inflammatories:

- Cayenne (*Capsicum annuum, C. frutescens*)
- Chamomile (*Matricaria recutita*)
- Rosemary (*Rosmarinus officinalis*)
- Sage (*Salvia officinalis, S. lavandulaefolia*)
- Tea (*Camellia sinensis*)
- Yarrow (*Achillea millefolium*)

Infection-Fighting Antimicrobials

Herbs with antimicrobial or antibiotic action destroy or inhibit the growth of disease-causing microorganisms like bacteria and viruses.

Herbal Antibiotics

Technically speaking, antibiotics are living cultures (like penicillin) or synthetic versions of live cultures that can kill or neutralize pathogens—in other words, they're not herbs. But several herbs have demonstrated an antibiotic-like effect in the body, making them viable options in the fight against infections.

ALERT!

Extracts of the mangosteen tree (*Garcinia mangostana*), used traditionally in Thailand and Sri Lanka as a remedy for diarrhea and skin infections, have been shown to be lethal to several strains of bacteria that are resistant to certain pharmaceutical antibiotics. That's big news today, as more and more disease-causing microbes are finding a way around antibiotic drugs.

Using herbs to fight microbial infections is a smart move. Research has shown that pharmaceutical germ-killers are overused and might contribute to the development and spread of drug-resistant microorganisms. What's more, even the best prescription antibiotics won't help a viral infection, as they're effective against bacteria only.

Antibiotics also carry lots of potential side effects, like stomach upset, headaches, and sensitivity to sunlight.

Antivirals, Antifungals, and Antibacterials

Herbs can treat viral infections like colds and flu, as well as coughs, cold sores, and sore throats. Herbal antifungals can combat yeast infections and other infections caused by fungi, such as athlete's foot. Antibacterial herbs are useful for treating bacterial skin infections and acne.

Many herbs can also combat infectious protozoa, single-celled organisms like *Cryptosporidium* or *Giardia* that can cause foodborne illness and diseases such as malaria. Here are some of the best-known antimicrobial herbs:

- Barberry (*Berberis vulgaris*)
- Elderberry (*Sambucus nigra*)
- Garlic (*Allium sativum*)
- Ginger (*Zingiber officinale*)
- Goldenseal (*Hydrastis canadensis*)
- Grape (*Vitis vinifera*)
- Rosemary (*Rosmarinus officinalis*)
- Tea tree (*Melaleuca alternifolia*)
- Thyme (*Thymus vulgaris*)

Herbal Antioxidants

Antioxidants have been the darling of the health media for several years now, and the studies demonstrating their disease-fighting powers continue to pile up. Research has also shown that plants—both edible fruits and vegetables and medicinal herbs—are the richest sources of antioxidant compounds.

An *antioxidant* is a molecule that can slow or prevent the oxidation of other molecules.

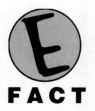

FACT

Many of the plants used as flavoring agents are also rich sources of antioxidants—even richer than the fruits and vegetables people have come to think of as disease-fighters. Case in point: Ounce for ounce, oregano (*Origanum vulgare*) delivers forty-two times more antioxidant activity than apples, twelve times more than oranges, and four times more than blueberries.

Oxidation is a natural chemical reaction that happens when one substance (known as an *oxidizing agent*) transfers electrons to another. It's a real paradox: Oxygen is crucial for survival, but it's a highly reactive element that can also cause problems.

Oxidation produces molecules called *free radicals*, which can damage cells through a process termed *oxidative stress*. And oxidative stress has been implicated in many diseases, including cancer and heart disease. Many plants—including medicinal herbs, culinary herbs, and plants eaten as food—are loaded with antioxidants. Some of the best-known plant-derived antioxidant compounds are:

- **Vitamin C** (in cayenne, citrus fruits, and walnuts)
- **Vitamin E** (in sunflower and flax oils)
- **Carotenoids** (in carrots and spinach)
- **Polyphenols like resveratrol** (in blueberries, grapes, and peanuts) **and flavonoids** (in citrus fruits, chocolate, and tea)

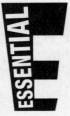

Flavonoids are a type of chemical compound called *phenols*, which are manufactured by plants as part of their self-defense system. Flavonoids are antioxidants that the plant synthesizes in response to oxidative stress—and they make excellent antioxidants for you, too.

Here are some of the more popular antioxidant herbs, many of which are eaten as foods or used as flavorings:

- **Fennel** (*Foeniculum vulgare*)
- **Garlic** (*Allium sativum*)
- **Grape** (*Vitis vinifera*)
- **Grapefruit** (*Citrus paradisi*)
- **Pomegranate** (*Punica granatum*)
- **Turmeric** (*Curcuma longa*)

Herbs to Aid Digestion

Herbalists have a remedy for practically any digestive woe you could have, from indigestion and nausea to diarrhea and gas.

Digestives

Herbal medicine offers several options for improving overall digestion. These herbs, generally known as digestives, stimulate the production of digestive fluids and encourage regular elimination. The best-known digestive herbs include these:

- **Chamomile** (*Matricaria recutita*)
- **Cinnamon** (*Cinnamomum verum, C. aromaticum*)
- **Fennel** (*Foeniculum vulgare*)
- **Peppermint** (*Mentha x piperita*)
- **Pineapple** (*Ananas comosus*)

Carminatives

Another group of herbs are classified as carminatives, meaning they work to dispel gas and relieve cramping. Carminatives have antispasmodic (anticramping) action on the muscles in the gastrointestinal tract. Here are some of the better-known carminatives:

- **Barberry** (*Berberis vulgaris*)
- **Fennel** (*Foeniculum vulgare*)
- **Licorice** (*Glycyrrhiza glabra*)
- **Rosemary** (*Rosmarinus officinalis*)
- **Tea** (*Camellia sinensis*)

Anti-diarrheals

Herbal remedies for diarrhea slow the transit of fluids through your GI tract to return your digestion to its normal pace. They include:

- **Barberry** (*Berberis vulgaris*)
- **Bilberry** (*Vaccinium myrtillus*)
- **Fenugreek** (*Trigonella foenum-graecum*)
- **Juniper** (*Juniperus communis*)
- **Marshmallow** (*Althaea officinalis*)
- **Psyllium** (*Plantago ovata, P. psyllium*)
- **Sangre de grado** (*Croton lechleri*)

Antiemetics

A group of herbs known as antiemetics work to combat nausea and stop vomiting. Herbal remedies for nausea and vomiting include these:

- **American ginseng** (*Panax quinquefolius*)
- **Dill** (*Anethum graveolens*)
- **Ginger** (*Zingiber officinale*)
- **Mate** (*Ilex paraguariensis*)
- **Tea** (*Camellia sinensis*)

Herbal demulcents soothe inflammation in the digestive tract:

- Alfalfa (*Medicago sativa*)
- Flax (*Linum usitatissimum*)
- Gentian (*Gentiana lutea*)

- Licorice (*Glycyrrhiza glabra*)
- Marshmallow (*Althaea officinalis*)

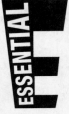

Herbs can also stimulate regurgitation. Ipecac (*Cephaelis ipecacuanha*) has been used by generations of indigenous people in the Amazon to induce vomiting. It was adopted by seventeenth-century Europeans and used to make syrup of ipecac, an OTC emetic and once-popular remedy for accidental poisoning.

Laxatives and Diuretics

Several medicinal plants aid in the elimination of bodily waste. Herbal purgatives (or laxatives) have been used for centuries to relieve constipation and speed the transit of food through the digestive system; diuretics are used to relieve water retention and treat high blood pressure (hypertension) and urinary tract infections. Herbal laxatives include:

- Aloe (*Aloe vera*)
- Flax (*Linum usitatissimum*)

- Fenugreek (*Trigonella foenum-graecum*)
- Psyllium (*Plantago ovata, P. psyllium*)

Some popular herbal diuretics are:

- Alfalfa (*Medicago sativa*)
- Dandelion (*Taraxacum officinale*)

- Nettle (*Urtica dioica*)
- Tea (*Camellia sinensis*)

Natural Cough Relief

Many herbs can function as natural cough syrups, aiding in the elimination of mucus and phlegm from the airways.

As with many medications, herbal options trump the pharmaceuticals in this area, as well, because they lack most of the side effects (and safety concerns) associated with the drugs.

In most cases, the herbs used as expectorants are safe for anyone out of diapers—something that can't be said for OTC expectorants, which the Food and Drug Administration doesn't recommend for anyone under the age of eleven. The FDA recently announced that it's looking into the matter after a spate of accidents involving kids and cough syrup.

Herbal Expectorants

Doctors recommend using an expectorant to help rid yourself of phlegm—you use it to help along a "productive" cough. Some herbal expectorants are:

- **Ginger** (*Zingiber officinale*)
- **Licorice** (*Glycyrrhiza glabra*)
- **Peppermint** (*Mentha x piperita*)
- **Rosemary** (*Rosmarinus officinalis*)

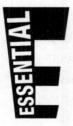

Before scientists developed the drugs used in today's cold and flu remedies, herbs like barberry (*Berberis vulgaris*), goldenseal (*Hydrastis canadensis*), ginkgo (*Ginkgo biloba*), rosemary (*Rosmarinus officinalis*), eleuthero (*Eleutherococcus senticosus*), and fennel (*Foeniculum vulgare*) were the remedies of choice for fighting coughs and other cold and flu symptoms.

Cough Suppressants

Antitussives are agents that suppress the urge to cough, and they're used when you've got a dry, painful cough that's not producing any phlegm. Some herbal options include:

- **Fennel** (*Foeniculum vulgare*)
- **Hops** (*Humulus lupulus*)
- **Licorice** (*Glycyrrhiza glabra*)
- **Marshmallow** (*Althaea officinalis*)
- **Spearmint** (*Mentha spicata*)

Sedatives and Stimulants

For centuries, herbalists have been using plants with sedating effects on the central nervous system to help treat insomnia and, in low doses, to relieve anxiety. At the same time, they've used an assortment of stimulating herbs, which boost mental and physical performance and fight fatigue.

ALERT!

Plants are almost always a better choice than any OTC or prescription drugs that work on the central nervous system—either sedatives or stimulants—because they generally don't carry the same side effects, which include agitation or excessive sedation, diarrhea or constipation, dizziness, hallucinations, and dependency.

Herbal stimulants work on the central nervous system, subtly increasing metabolic processes to increase alertness and energy.

Herbal Sleep Aids

Plant-based sedatives can be tailored to your specific needs—the herbs used to treat insomnia and agitation vary widely in their sedating effect—and in most cases you can mix them with other remedies (or a glass of wine) without worrying about drug interaction. Here are some of the most popular herbal sedatives:

- Chamomile (*Matricaria recutita*)
- Kava (*Piper methysticum*)
- Lavender (*Lavandula angustifolia*)
- Lemon balm (*Melissa officinalis*)
- Passionflower (*Passiflora incarnata*)
- Valerian (*Valeriana officinalis*)

Herbs That Stimulate

Stimulant herbs can provide a gentle boost to your mental and physical energy levels. Here are some of the better-known herbal stimulants:

- Asian ginseng (*Panax ginseng*)
- Cocoa (*Theobroma cacao*)
- Coffee (*Coffea arabica*)
- Guarana (*Paullinia cupana*)
- Mate (*Ilex paraguariensis*)
- Tea (*Camellia sinensis*)

Mood Boosters

Many herbs have proven psychiatric effects, meaning they can relieve depression, anxiety, and other psychological disorders the same way that pharmaceuticals can. The big advantage of herbal antidepressants and anxiety remedies is the fact that they're almost entirely free of side effects—something that no lab-created drug can promise.

Consider the most commonly prescribed antidepressants, like sertraline (Zoloft) and citalopram hydrobromide (Celexa), which are part of the class of drugs known as *selective serotonin reuptake inhibitors*, or SSRIs. The most common side effects of these medications are nausea, diarrhea, headaches, and sexual dysfunction.

And while quality research on herbal depression and anxiety remedies is still slim, several studies have shown that herbal remedies like Saint John's wort (*Hypericum perforatum*) can work as well as prescription medications in cases of mild to moderate depression.

Herbs can alter the levels of the neurotransmitters *serotonin* and *dopamine*, which are central in depression and other mood disorders as well as addictions and other psychological problems. Here are some herbs with mood-lifting effects:

- **Boswellia** (*Boswellia serrata*)
- **Lemon balm** (*Melissa officinalis*)
- **Passionflower** (*Passiflora incarnata*)
- **Rhodiola** (*Rhodiola rosea*)
- **Saint John's wort** (*Hypericum perforatum*)

These herbs have been used successfully to treat anxiety:

- **Ashwagandha** (*Withania somnifera*)
- **Chamomile** (*Matricaria recutita*)
- **Hops** (*Humulus lupulus*)
- **Kava** (*Piper methysticum*)
- **Lavender** (*Lavandula angustifolia*)
- **Lemon balm** (*Melissa officinalis*)

These herbs can be used to treat addictions and eating disorders:

- **Danshen** (*Salvia miltiorrhiza*)
- **Ginkgo** (*Ginkgo biloba*)
- **Kudzu** (*Pueraria lobata*)
- **Passionflower** (*Passiflora incarnata*)
- **Saint John's wort** (*Hypericum perforatum*)

CHAPTER 3

Herbs for Women

Quite often the symptoms and treatments of certain health conditions vary enormously between the genders, and men and women typically manage their health concerns very differently. In addition, several important health problems, including depression, osteoarthritis, chronic fatigue syndrome, osteoporosis, and autoimmune diseases, are significantly more common in women than in men.

Women Are Different

Most often, women are physically smaller—they weigh less and have smaller organs, less muscle mass, and more body fat—than men. Women also produce less of certain chemicals, such as those that synthesize the brain chemical serotonin (which plays a big role in depression and other mood disorders, as well as appetite and eating habits).

While men and women perform equally on intelligence tests, women's brains have more gray matter (the part that allows thinking) and less white matter (the part that transfers information among various regions). This may explain why women seem to be better at verbal and memory challenges, while men excel at spatial tasks.

Many of the differences in health concerns can be traced to hormones. For example, research has shown that female sex hormones might be related to the development and progression of allergies and asthma, both of which are more prevalent in women. Estrogen, the best known of the women's hormones, has been linked to women's greater susceptibility to lung cancer as well as the "hormonal cancers" that include breast and ovarian cancer.

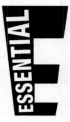

Migraines strike women far more often than men. In any given year, roughly 18 percent of women over the age of twelve will experience at least one, compared to about 6 or 7 percent of men. Experts think that hormones—and hormonal fluctuations—are responsible for the gender discrepancy.

Hormones can partly be blamed for women's greater sensitivity to pain and to stimulants like cocaine and amphetamines. This sensitivity also fluctuates with a woman's menstrual cycle. Hormones might explain why women often react differently than men to anesthesia (women wake up more quickly but are more prone to side effects such as post-operative vomiting or nausea).

Herbs for Women's Health

Women have been relying on herbal medicines for centuries, and more women than men turn to herbs today. Recent surveys indicate that 79 percent of U.S. women take herbal medicines. Statistics also show that women are much more likely to take charge of their own health—they see their primary physician regularly and typically act on medical concerns instead of ignoring them. Women are also more likely to try a novel or unconventional type of health care treatment, both to treat a specific condition as well as to promote general well being.

Natural Estrogens

Many medicinal and edible plants contain compounds called *phytoestrogens*, which are chemically similar to the sex hormone estradiol (the primary estrogen in humans). Estradiol is critical to many body processes, including reproduction, sexual functioning, the synthesis of bone, and the modulation of several diseases (including cancer and heart disease). Phytoestrogens seem to modulate estrogen levels in the body, which can cause a host of beneficial effects and may avert certain diseases.

Many of the so-called women's herbs contain a group of phytoestrogens known as isoflavones, which are found in soy (*Glycine max*). Another type, lignans, are found in soy and flax (*Linum usitatissimum*). A third type, coumestans, is found in red clover (*Trifolium pratense*) and alfalfa (*Medicago sativa*).

Research has linked phytoestrogen intake with many health benefits, including preventing osteoporosis, managing cholesterol, and reducing the risk of some cancers.

However, consuming excessive amounts can cause problems. Experts suggest sticking to recommended doses of herbal remedies and eating a sensible amount of phytoestrogen-containing foods (like soy). See Chapter 18 for more.

Using Herbs Wisely

Following are some tips for women on using herbal preparations.

- **Talk with Your Doctor.** Be sure to tell your doctor about any herbs you're considering, especially if you're pregnant or are being treated for a serious and/or chronic condition.

- **Don't Assume That "Natural" Means "Good."** Herbal medicines are considered supplements—or foods—and not drugs, so they're handled much differently than pharmaceuticals. The Food and Drug Administration (FDA) doesn't require that the manufacturer prove an herb's safety, quality, or efficacy. This certainly doesn't mean that all supplements are suspect, just that you should use them with care.

- **Know Your Body.** Everyone responds differently to chemical agents, whether they're from a plant or a pharmacy, so different people will require different doses. If you know you're sensitive to medications, start with a very small dose of the herbal preparation. Even if you're not overly sensitive, you should never exceed the recommended dosage.

- **Pay Attention.** Most herbs have very low risk of interactions or side effects, but you should monitor yourself when starting any new therapy.

- **Be Patient.** Most herbal remedies take a bit longer to produce effects than prescription or over-the-counter (OTC) medicines do. Most experts advise patients to allow several weeks before deciding if a remedy is working or not, and note that some herbs may take up to eight weeks to deliver any benefits.

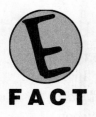

FACT

Gamma-linolenic acid, or GLA, supports immune, endocrine (hormonal), and cardiovascular functioning and is used to treat several women's health issues, including menstrual and menopausal symptoms. The best-known herbal source is evening primrose (*Oenothera biennis*) oil, which can be expensive. Other good sources of GLAs are borage (*Borago officinalis*) and black currant (*Ribes nigrum*) oils.

Breast Health

The breasts are made up of several types of tissue: glandular tissue (including mammary glands that produce milk and ducts that transport it), connective tissue, and fat. Breast tissue changes throughout a woman's life, with menstrual cycles as well as general aging.

Breast Pain

Breast pain, also known as mastalgia, is fairly common, affecting about 70 percent of women at some point in their lives. Severe mastaglia, which occurs more than five days a month and can be quite debilitating, affects about 10 percent of women.

Breast pain can be cyclic (changing with the menstrual cycle) and noncyclic (constant or intermittent pain that's not tied to your period). Cyclic pain, which is the most common, typically affects both breasts and involves dull pain, swelling, tenderness, and lumpiness in the entire breast. Noncyclic breast pain is more common in postmenopausal women, usually affects just one breast, and is localized.

Although the exact causes of breast pain aren't known, most experts think that cyclic pain is tied to hormonal fluctuations, while noncyclic pain is caused by physical factors such as breast cysts (see below) or trauma. Taking oral contraceptives, menopause treatments, and antidepressants has also been tied to breast pain. Some experts think it might be tied to an imbalance of fatty acids like gamma-linolenic acid (GLA), which makes the breast tissue more sensitive to hormonal changes (and pain).

Lumps and Bumps

Lumps in the breast can be caused by many things—some dangerous, most benign. In the majority of cases, a lump is a harmless swelling or thickening of tissue caused by a group of conditions termed *fibrocystic breast changes* (FCCs), which affect at least half of all women, most often between the ages of twenty and fifty. FCCs include fibrosis, which is the development of fibrous tissue, and cysts, which are small sacs created when an overgrowth of tissue blocks the milk ducts and causes the glands to fill with fluid. Cysts are typically smooth, with defined edges, and feel like small, soft grapes; they can occur singly or in groups. Breast cysts generally disappear after menopause. One exception: Postmenopausal women taking hormone replacement therapy (HRT), which can trigger the formation of cysts.

Cysts can get to be one or two inches in diameter, and larger cysts can put pressure on surrounding tissues, causing pain. In most cases, cysts will resolve themselves without any treatment, although doctors can drain the fluid from large cysts that have become uncomfortable.

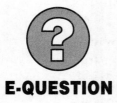

E-QUESTION

Does a lump in the breast always mean cancer?
Finding a lump is rarely a sign of cancer, but if you notice a mass in your breast that doesn't go away after one menstrual period and/or is accompanied by other symptoms, such as redness or changes in breast shape or skin texture, you should schedule an appointment with your doctor. Localized pain that doesn't change with your menstrual cycle also warrants an exam.

Drug (and Nondrug) Treatments

Most doctors recommend OTC pain medications such as nonsteroidal anti-inflammatory drugs (NSAIDs) to treat breast pain. In severe cases, prescription medicines might be prescribed, such as danazol (Danazol), which is a synthetic steroid. NSAIDs can cause gastrointestinal damage and other side effects, and danazol can cause acne and unwanted hair growth.

Herbalists offer a few natural approaches to breast pain and fibrocystic breast changes:

- **Evening primrose** (*Oenothera biennis*)   The seeds of this flowering plant contain gamma-linolenic acid (GLA), which is a valuable anti-inflammatory. Evening primrose oil has been shown to reduce both cyclic and noncyclic breast pain.

- **Red clover** (*Trifolium pratense*)   Red clover is a traditional remedy for cyclic mastalgia. Recent research has shown that an extract of the herb significantly reduces breast pain and tenderness in nearly half the women who try it.

- **Vitex** (*Vitex agnus-castus*)   Vitex seems to have estrogenic activity in the body and has been shown to relieve cyclic breast pain.

Menstrual Issues

Menstruation, or menses, is the cyclical process that women go through roughly once a month from around age fourteen to age fifty. During menstruation, the uterus sheds its lining (the endometrium) through the vagina. In most cases, it's a fairly uneventful process. But for some women, menstruation can bring serious discomfort.

PMS, or premenstrual syndrome, occurs in the week or two weeks before a woman's menstrual period and generally stops as soon as menstruation begins. PMS affects about 75 percent of women. Common symptoms are breast tenderness, acne, insomnia, headache and backache, tension, and irritability. PMS is tied to changing hormone levels and can be exacerbated by stress.

About 8 percent of women experience a particularly severe form of PMS known as premenstrual dysphoric disorder (PMDD), which is a serious, often debilitating condition that can include marked depression, anger, flu-like symptoms, and appetite and sleep changes.

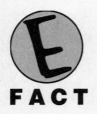

FACT

Stress affects everyone, but it can be especially tough on women (and trigger PMS and other problems). The American Psychological Association reports that mothers in the "sandwich generation" (ages thirty-five to fifty-four) feel more stress than any other group. And while two out of every five Americans say they feel overextended, more women than men report extreme stress.

Treatment of PMS generally includes OTC medicines like Midol, which contain an NSAID or other pain reliever, plus a diuretic to fight bloating. Women with PMDD are often given antidepressants as well.

Serious menstrual cramps, also known as dysmenorrhea, can strike at any age, although teenagers are more likely to have painful periods than older women. Postmenopausal cramps warrant a doctor's visit, as they can be caused by endometriosis, a painful condition in which tissue similar to that in the endometrium is found elsewhere in the body.

Many women treat the cramps and other symptoms of dysmenorrhea with OTC pain medications. In severe cases, doctors may prescribe oral contraceptives. Herbal remedies for premenstrual and menstrual problems include the following:

- **Dandelion** (*Taraxacum officinale*)

  Dandelion is a traditional remedy for the water retention of PMS. It's an herbal diuretic (it increases urine volume and sodium excretion to relieve bloating). Juniper (*Juniperus communis*) is another bloat-relieving option.

- **Ginkgo** (*Ginkgo biloba*)

  Ginkgo, better known for its memory-boosting benefits, can also relieve the moodiness and breast tenderness of PMS.

- **Maritime pine** (*Pinus pinaster*)

  Extracts of the bark from this French pine tree have been shown to relieve the pain of menstrual cramps and endometriosis.

- **Saint John's wort** (*Hypericum perforatum*)

  This mood-lifter has been shown to improve symptoms of PMS by as much as 50 percent; it's also effective against PMDD.

- **Vitex** (*Vitex agnus-castus*)

  Clinical trials show that vitex can reduce the psychological symptoms of both PMS and PMDD (its effects are comparable to the drug Prozac). It's also effective at relieving physical symptoms like headaches, water retention, and acne.

Female-Specific Infections

Because of their anatomy, women are prone to a few infections that seldom, if ever, strike men. Women also can blame their susceptibility to certain infections on their hormones.

UTIs

Urinary tract infections (UTIs) are about fifty times more common in women than in men, mostly because a woman has a shorter urethra (the tube that carries urine from the body), meaning bacteria have a shorter distance to travel in order to establish themselves in the bladder. Sexual activity—especially if you're using a diaphragm or spermicide—as well as douching, taking long baths, or holding urine for long periods of time all can increase your risk of UTIs.

If you think you've got a UTI, schedule a visit to the doctor right away. Conventional treatment almost always includes antibiotics, such as trimethoprim-sulfamethoxazole (Bactrim, Septra) or ciprofloxacin (Cipro).

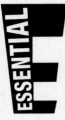

The most common type of UTI is *cystitis*, which affects the lower urinary tract. Symptoms include increased urinary frequency, urgency (the desire to urinate), and painful urination. Infections of the upper urinary tract, called pyelonephritis, are much more serious because they involve the kidney. Symptoms can include chills, fever, nausea, and internal pain.

Vaginal Infections

Bacterial vaginosis is characterized by watery vaginal discharge with an unpleasant odor, sometimes accompanied by burning, itching, or redness. It's caused by an overgrowth of bacteria, which can be aided by wearing tight, nonbreathable clothing, douching, and using "feminine deodorant" sprays. Conventional treatment typically involves antibiotics like metronidazole (Flagyl).

A vaginal yeast infection, also known as *candidiasis*, is caused by an overgrowth of an organism called *Candida albicans*. *Candida* infections show up in other parts of the body, as well: Thrush (which affects the mouth and throat), jock itch, and athlete's foot are examples. Most of the time, *Candida* yeasts live in body without any problem but can trigger symptoms if their numbers get out of control.

Yeast infections are characterized by sticky white or yellowish discharge, burning, and itching. They're fairly common—nearly 75 percent of adult women will have at least one episode in her lifetime—but occur more frequently and more severely in people with weakened immune systems.

Overuse of broad-spectrum antibiotics, which kill off the so-called "good" bacteria that keep yeast under control, has been implicated in candidiasis, as have corticosteroid drugs and high-sugar diets.

Conventional medicine treats candidiasis with antifungal drugs, including suppositories and topical creams like miconazole (Monistat) and single-dose oral medications such as fluconazole (Diflucan).

Herbal Alternatives

UTIs can be treated with the following herbs:

- **Cranberry** (*Vaccinium macrocarpon*)

  Cranberry juice is rich in antioxidants and one of the best-known natural remedies for urinary tract infections. Lab tests show that it prevents bacteria from adhering to the tissues in the urinary tract. Blueberry (*Vaccinium angustifolium*) juice and extract contain similar chemicals.

- **Dandelion** (*Taraxacum officinale*)

  Research shows that a combination of dandelion and uva ursi (*Arctostaphylos uva-ursi, Arbutus uva-ursi*) can reduce the incidence of UTIs.

- **Juniper** (*Juniperus communis*)

  Juniper extracts are antibacterial and stimulate the flow of urine. Juniper berries were a standard treatment for UTIs for several Native American tribes.

Herbal remedies for bacterial vaginosis and candidiasis include:

- **Echinacea** (*Echinacea purpurea*)

  This classic immune-boosting herb can help pharmaceuticals do their job even better. Recent research has shown that echinacea extracts can boost the effectiveness of antifungal drugs in treating candidiasis.

- **Goldenseal** (*Hydrastis canadensis*)

  This herb is a powerful antibacterial and antifungal and can be taken orally or used topically to fight bacterial vaginitis or candidiasis. Goldenseal's infection-fighting powers have been attributed in large part to the chemical berberine, which is also plentiful in barberry (*Berberis vulgaris*).

- **Tea tree** (*Melaleuca alternifolia*)

  Known for its antibacterial and antifungal properties, this Australian import has been shown in several studies to eradicate both the bacteria and the yeast cells responsible for vaginal infections when applied topically or used as a douche.

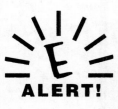
ALERT!

The ready availability of OTC antifungal remedies has made it much easier for women to treat vaginal candidiasis themselves, but these medications are often misused. According to the Centers for Disease Control and Prevention, as many as two-thirds of the OTC drugs sold to treat vaginal candidiasis were used by women who didn't actually have a *Candida* infection, a habit that can lead to the development of drug-resistant infections.

Sexual Health and Fertility

Being sexually healthy—having an interest in sex, being able to function sexually, and being able to get pregnant (if she so chooses)—is a key part of a woman's overall well being.

A woman's sexual desire, or libido, can go up and down naturally, for many different reasons (and usually for a short time). However, sex drive that's perpetually stuck in neutral deserves attention. Some medications, notably antidepressants, can cause a drop in libido, as can shifts in hormone levels and changes in sleep patterns and stress levels.

Most women can expect to be fertile—capable of getting pregnant—for the full extent of their reproductive years (the time between the first menses and the onset of menopause). A woman is considered "infertile" if she and her partner have been trying for a year to get pregnant (and her partner's fertility has been verified by a doctor).

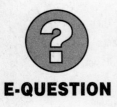

E-QUESTION

Can herbs work as contraceptives?
Several herbs traditionally used to prevent pregnancy are now being seriously studied for more widespread use. For example, the Indian herb neem (*Azadirachta indica*) works as a safe and reversible contraceptive. In one study, rats given an intrauterine shot of neem were infertile for up to 180 days, then had healthy litters with no apparent problems.

Female infertility can be caused by a physical problem (such as ovarian cysts or a blocked fallopian tube), a hormonal imbalance, or various other factors (such as age, stress, or poor nutrition). In most cases, it's a temporary condition.

Conventional and Other Approaches

Conventional medicine typically addresses women's sexual irregularities with things like counseling and stress reduction. Fertility treatments typically include drugs that stimulate ovulation, such as follicle-stimulating hormone, or FSH (Follistim), which can cause pulmonary and vascular problems and other side effects. Other options include *in vitro* fertilization. Here are some herbs that can help:

- **Ashwagandha** (*Withania somnifera*)

  Ashwagandha is considered a sexual stimulant for both men and women in Ayurvedic tradition, as is the herb schisandra (*Schisandra chinensis*). Both appear to increase sensitivity in the genitals (and thus stimulate the libido).

- **Rhodiola** (*Rhodiola rosea*)

  Rhodiola seems to restore fertility to women who have minor hormonal imbalances or are suffering the effects of stress.

- **Shatavari** (*Asparagus racemosus*)

  Shatavari, which means—no kidding—"she who has hundreds of husbands" in Sanskrit, is used in Ayurvedic medicine to increase sexual vitality and fertility.

- **Vitex** (*Vitex agnus-castus*)

  Research has shown that vitex can increase a woman's chance of getting pregnant.

- **Yohimbe** (*Pausinystalia yohimbe*)

  Yohimbe is an African herb used as an aphrodisiac and sexual function treatment for both men and women. In women, it seems to work by dilating vaginal blood vessels to increase circulation.

Pregnancy

Pregnancy can be a time of chaos for many women: They're experiencing any number of new sensations (and discomforts)—and they're worried about putting anything even potentially dangerous into their bodies.

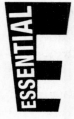

Stretch marks—small, raised marks that develop on the skin in areas that are experiencing rapid growth—are a concern for many pregnant women. Gotu kola (*Centella asiatica*), an Ayurvedic herb known for its ability to speed healing and reduce scarring, can help, as can ultramoisturizing cocoa (*Theobroma cacao*) butter and almond (*Prunus dulcis*) and sesame (*Sesamum indicum*) oils.

In many ways, pregnant women are the toughest group of people to treat—both conventionally and herbally—because so little is known about the effects of various compounds on the developing fetus.

Nausea, or morning sickness, is a common complaint during pregnancy, especially in the first few months. Other pregnant women suffer from constipation, heartburn, gas, and bloating. Pregnant women are generally advised to skip the usual OTC remedies for nausea and other gastrointestinal problems. The good news is that herbal medicine has a few alternatives:

- **Ginger** (*Zingiber officinale*)

  Taking extracts (or drinking tea) made from gingerroot has been shown to reduce nausea and vomiting.

- **Peppermint** (*Mentha x piperita*)

  Peppermint tea is another classic remedy for pregnancy-related nausea (and inhaling peppermint oil can relieve headaches). Skip the peppermint if you've got heartburn, however, as it might make your symptoms worse.

- **Psyllium** (*Plantago ovata, P. psyllium*)

  The seeds of this plant are a safe and effective remedy for constipation and its attendant symptoms.

ALERT!

Many herbs—including several "women's herbs"—should be avoided during pregnancy. They include: red clover (*Trifolium pratense*), black cohosh (*Actaea racemosa, Cimicifuga racemosa*), dong quai (*Angelica sinensis*), feverfew (*Tanacetum parthenium*), kava (*Piper methysticum*), Saint John's wort (*Hypericum perforatum*), and vitex (*Vitex agnus-castus*), plus caffeine-containing herbs like mate (*Ilex paraguariensis*), guarana (*Paullinia cupana*), coffee (*Coffea arabica*), and tea (*Camellia sinensis*).

Pregnancy can bring on headaches, backaches, and other kinds of aches—yet pregnant women are generally told to avoid NSAIDs and other pain-relieving pharmaceuticals. Happily, there are some herbal alternatives:

- **Cayenne** (*Capsicum annuum, C. frutescens*)

  These peppers contain the chemical capsaicin, which has been shown to reduce muscle pain and headaches when applied topically.

- **Maritime pine** (*Pinus pinaster*)

  Pine extracts have been shown to reduce the incidence of lower back pain, hip joint pain, pelvic pain, and pain due to varicose veins or calf cramps.

- **Witch hazel** (*Hamamelis virginiana*)

  Witch hazel can reduce the swelling, itching, and discomfort of hemorrhoids.

Menopause

The transition between fertility and menopause is technically known as perimenopause (or climacteric), but most people simply call it menopause. Menopause is the end of menses, and it's official when a woman hasn't had a period for twelve consecutive months. The average age of menopause is fifty-one, but anything between forty-one and fifty-nine is considered normal.

Symptoms

Menopause produces a few distinct symptoms, all the result of the shortfall in the hormones estrogen and progesterone created when the ovaries stop producing them.

ALERT!

The best-known menopause drug, Premarin, contains conjugated estrogens taken from the urine of pregnant female horses (its name is an abbreviation of "pregnant mares' urine"). Despite its side effects (including cramping, bloating, breast pain, hair loss, irregular bleeding, and *Candida* infections) and protests against the inhumane treatment of the "donor" mares, it's still routinely prescribed by conventional doctors.

These symptoms, which can go on for as little as a few weeks or as long as a few years, vary greatly among women. The most common include:

Vasomotor Symptoms

Menopausal vasomotor symptoms—those involving constriction or dilation of blood vessels—include hot flashes and night sweats.

Hot flashes are the most common symptom of menopause; almost all menopausal women have them. They are marked by a warm sensation that travels from your chest up into your head, often in waves, accompanied by a flushing in your skin and, in some cases, dizziness, nausea, headache, and rapid heartbeat. Hot flashes that come on at night are called *night sweats* (for obvious reasons).

Emotional and Cognitive Changes

Many women experience changes in mood—including depression and anxiety—during menopause. Other problems, like difficulty with concentration or memory, are also common.

Help for Menopausal Symptoms

Conventional medicine generally treats menopausal symptoms with hormone-like drugs that mimic the effects of estrogen and progesterone.

Until fairly recently, conventional doctors routinely prescribed the long-term use of drugs known as hormone replacement therapy (HRT) to both ease the symptoms of menopause and protect postmenopausal women against estrogen-mediated diseases like osteoporosis, Alzheimer's disease, and cardiovascular disease.

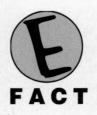

FACT

Insomnia is a common complaint among menopausal women. But several herbs used in aromatherapy (and inhaled or applied to the skin via massage), including lavender (*Lavandula angustifolia*) and jasmine (*Jasminum officinale*), can help you get to sleep without the side effects of pharmaceutical sedatives.

But recent research has shown that HRT actually increases the risk of cardiovascular problems (including stroke and heart attack), breast cancer, gall bladder disease, and dementia. These days, doctors usually prescribe HRT only for the short-term relief of menopausal symptoms.

However, even when it's used for a limited time, HRT has its side effects, including bloating, weight gain, and emotional problems like irritability and depression. But herbalism has a few alternatives:

- **Black cohosh** (*Actaea racemosa, Cimicifuga racemosa*) — Black cohosh extracts can significantly reduce hot flashes (one study showed an effect similar to a pharmaceutical estradiol patch).

- **Dong quai** (*Angelica sinensis*) — In a recent study, menopausal women who took a combination of dong quai and chamomile (*Matricaria recutita*) showed significant improvement in hot flashes.

- **Flax**
  (*Linum usitatissimum*)

  Taking flaxseed has been shown to reduce mild menopausal symptoms just as well as hormone therapy—without the side effects.

- **Kava**
  (*Piper methysticum*)

  Research has shown that kava extracts can reduce symptoms of anxiety and cognitive impairment in menopausal women—and results were seen after just one week.

- **Kudzu**
  (*Pueraria lobata*)

  Extracts of this Chinese vine, which is a traditional Chinese menopause treatment, seem to improve cognitive function in postmenopausal women.

- **Red clover**
  (*Trifolium pratense*)

  Red clover is a traditional remedy for menopausal complaints, and there is some evidence that it can reduce hot flashes, lower cholesterol levels, and improve cognitive functioning.

- **Soy**
  (*Glycine max*)

  Soy—both the dietary and the supplemental kind—can decrease the severity and frequency of hot flashes. In some studies, the effects were similar to those of pharmaceutical hormone therapy.

- **Saint John's wort**
  (*Hypericum perforatum*)

  Research shows that a combination of Saint John's wort and black cohosh (*Actaea racemosa, Cimicifuga racemosa*) can reduce depression and other psychological symptoms of menopause.

CHAPTER 4

Herbs for Men

Some male issues overlap with female concerns—both genders face chronic conditions like heart disease, diabetes, and many cancers, as well as issues of general wellness like sexual functioning, fitness and exercise, skin and hair care—but men also have issues that are theirs alone. And quite often, diseases strike men in a different way, producing a separate set of symptoms and demanding distinct prevention and treatment strategies.

Men Are Different

Because of their physical structure and hormonal chemistry, men face a unique group of health concerns. The good news is that many of them can be treated safely and effectively with herbal remedies.

The most obvious differences between the sexes lie in their reproductive systems. But there are other variables, too. Men are, for the most part, physically bigger than women—they're taller, with a bigger skeleton (made up of denser, stronger bones), more muscle mass and body fat, thicker skin, and bigger organs. Men also have a higher metabolic rate. They generally sweat more, and they have greater heart and lung capacity.

Even before they're born, males and females are exposed to the sex hormones that will define them for the rest of their lives. By the age of two, gender-specific physical characteristics start appearing, and as a child approaches puberty, they'll become more obvious.

In males, these traits are created in large part by the hormone testosterone, which is an androgen, or steroid, hormone produced in the testes and the principal male sex hormone. Among other things, testosterone works to increase the size of the boy's muscles and bones and, later on, to deepen his voice, change the shape of his skeleton (including the bones of his face), and promote the growth of facial and body hair.

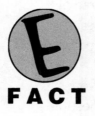

FACT

Hormones affect memory. Research shows that women remember more words, faces, and everyday events than men do, meaning a woman will probably remember a conversation in which she got the directions to a friend's house. Meanwhile, men can recall more symbolic, nonlinguistic information, meaning the man will be better at navigation when it comes to finding his way home again.

As adults, male and female hormones play a big role in health and the development of disease. For example, in women, estradiol levels have been tied to the perception of pain, the development of allergies and asthma, and the initiation and progression of certain cancers. In men, testosterone is related to cardiac and sexual functioning, immunity and response to injury, and the building and maintenance of bone and muscle. It also seems to play a role in prostate health and obesity.

Men's Herbalism

All of the world's schools of herbal medicine have treatments and remedies specifically for men. For example, Traditional Chinese Medicine (TCM) views sexual dysfunction in men as a loss of *yang*, or primary life force, which is stored in the kidneys. It's therefore treated with kidney-warming herbs like schisandra (*Schisandra chinensis*) and epimedium (*Epimedium sagittatum*). Meanwhile, Western herbalists treated impotence with circulation-boosting herbs like cinnamon (*Cinnamomum verum, C. aromaticum*) and clove (*Syzygium aromaticum*).

Herbal Hormones

Many medicinal and edible plants contain compounds called *phytoestrogens*, which are chemically similar to the sex hormone estradiol, the primary estrogen in humans. Although it's generally regarded as a "woman's hormone," estradiol also occurs naturally in a man's body (it's produced in the testes). In addition, as in a woman's body, a man's body produces precursor hormones (including testosterone), which are converted to estradiol. In a man's body, estradiol is involved in sexual functioning, the synthesis of bone, cognitive functioning, and the modulation of several diseases (including cancer and heart disease).

Most phytoestrogens are a type of plant chemical known as isoflavones; the best-known source is soy (*Glycine max*). Another kind of phytoestrogens, lignans, are in flax (*Linum usitatissimum*). A third type, coumestans, can be found red clover (*Trifolium pratense*) and alfalfa (*Medicago sativa*).

In men, dietary phytoestrogens have been associated with lower rates of prostate cancer. However, men should avoid consuming excessive amounts, as some studies have shown that soy intake can reduce a man's sperm count (other studies have had different results, meaning the jury is still out on the question).

To be safe, men should avoid medicinal herbs that are high in phytoestrogens and stick to sensible amounts of soy and other phytoestrogen-containing foods.

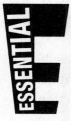

Estrogen, like any other hormone, can be both beneficial and harmful. Research has shown that a few chemicals, called *estrogenic xenobiotics*, can mimic estrogen in the body and cause health problems the same way that excessive estrogen might do naturally. For example, the chemical nonylphenol, found in cleaning products, paints, herbicides, and pesticides, can damage human sperm.

Using Herbs Wisely

Here are some tips for men on using herbs and preparations:

- **Keep Your Doctor Informed.** Talk with your doctor about any herbs you're considering, especially if you're being treated for a serious and/or chronic condition.
- **Do Your Homework.** "Natural" doesn't necessarily mean "good" (or even "safe"). Herbs are considered supplements—not drugs—and so are handled more like foods than pharmaceuticals. The Food and Drug Administration (FDA) doesn't require supplement manufacturers to prove an herb's safety, quality, or efficacy. So be sure to buy from reputable sources, and always follow the manufacturer's guidelines.
- **Pay Attention.** Everyone responds differently to medicines, whether they're from a plant or a pharmacy, so everyone requires a different dose. This is especially true with herbs, which can vary significantly in potency from one product to another. Most herbs have very low risk of interactions or side effects, but you should monitor yourself when starting any new therapy.
- **Give It Time.** Most herbal remedies take a bit longer to produce effects than pharmaceuticals do. Experts advise allowing several weeks before deciding if a remedy is working for you.

Sexual Functioning

Male sexual difficulties involve getting or keeping an erection, ejaculating too rapidly, having difficulty reaching orgasm, or failing to impregnate a woman after regular unprotected sex (see "Fertility and Infertility," below). Most men experience these problems at some time or another, but if a problem is chronic, a man (and his partner) will want some answers.

In the United States, roughly half of all men over fifty—as many as 30 million individuals—have some degree of *erectile dysfunction*, or ED (also called impotence). ED is the repeated inability to get or keep an erection firm enough for sexual intercourse, and chronic ED affects about one in five American men.

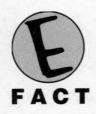

FACT

Erectile dysfunction can be caused by many things, including age (it's fairly common in men over sixty-five) and the use of some drugs (including depression and blood pressure medications). It's also associated with obesity, smoking, and high cholesterol, as well as certain diseases (as many as 80 percent of diabetic men develop ED).

Conventional treatments for ED most often include the prescription drugs sildenafil citrate (Viagra), vardenafil (Levitra), and tadalafil (Cialis). Another option is the drug alprostadil (Caverject), which you inject directly into your penis or insert, in pellet form, into your urethra. Doctors also prescribe mechanical vacuum devices and, in some cases, will surgically implant a prosthetic. Needless to say, each of these options has its own set of drawbacks and potential side effects. For example, sildenafil has been associated with serious cardiovascular and nervous system problems and priapism (prolonged, painful erections), as well as more minor side effects such as headache and excessive sweating.

Two other common sexual difficulties in men include premature ejaculation and low libido. Premature ejaculation happens when a man reaches orgasm during intercourse sooner than he or his partner wishes. Low libido is a case of lower-than-normal (or lower-than-desired) sex drive. Both are caused most often by psychological stress or anxiety.

Herbal remedies for ED, ejaculation problems, and low libido include:

- **Asian ginseng** (*Panax ginseng*)

  This is a classic remedy for impotence. Modern studies show that Asian ginseng extracts can improve symptoms of ED.

- **Ginkgo** (*Ginkgo biloba*)

  Ginkgo is known to improve circulation throughout the body, which might help with ED (it also contains the amino acid arginine, which can help relieve impotence). Ginkgo extracts also can reduce the sexual side effects of certain antidepressant drugs.

- **Kava** (*Piper methysticum*)

  Kava root can be used to increase sex drive. It's been shown to directly affect brain chemistry, instilling a sense of well being and alleviating the anxiety that can lead to sexual dysfunction.

- **Maca** (*Lepidium meyenii*)

  Extracts of this hardy Peruvian plant have been proven to increase sexual desire in otherwise healthy men.

- **Maritime pine** (*Pinus pinaster*)

  Pine bark extracts can improve sexual functioning in men with ED.

- **Yohimbe** (*Pausinystalia yohimbe*)

  Research has shown that extracts of the bark of this African evergreen are effective treatments for male sexual dysfunction and impotence and can treat ED that's caused by structural, circulatory, and psychological problems.

Fertility and Infertility

For many men, fathering a child is an important, almost essential, part of life, so problems related to fertility can be extremely distressing. Infertility is defined as the condition in which a sexually active couple has had difficulty getting pregnant for several months or longer.

A difficulty in fertility is referred to as "male factor" infertility if it is traced to a problem with the man's sperm—either there aren't enough, they are damaged in some way, or they're having a problem with motility (the ability to move freely and spontaneously).

Depending on the diagnosis, conventional medical treatments for male factor infertility can involve drugs (antibiotics to treat an infection, for example), hormones (to treat low testosterone levels), or surgery (to treat a pituitary tumor or an enlargement of the veins in the scrotum, called *varicocele*).

If your doctor can't trace your problem to any of these conditions, you might want to try an herbal remedy that's known to boost male fertility.

- **Astragalus** (*Astragalus membranaceus*)

  This is a classic remedy in Chinese medicine for male factor infertility. Modern research has shown that extracts can enhance sperm motility.

- **Eleuthero** (*Eleutherococcus senticosus*)

  This herb, also known as Siberian ginseng, can enhance the body's response to stress (and thus can help with stress-related infertility problems). Research has shown that eleuthero extracts can enhance sperm motility.

- **Goji-berry** (*Lycium barbarum, L. chinense*)

  The fruits of the lycium plant, also known as wolfberries, are considered a tonic, or superior, medicine in Chinese herbalism and are used to treat impotence, sexual debility, and low sperm count (the plant is also known as matrimony vine). Modern research shows that goji-berry can improve sperm quantity and quality.

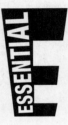

Male infertility can be tied to genetics, problems with your immune system, the use of some medications (including steroids, antihypertensives, antidepressants, and anticancer drugs), chronic infection, hormone disorders (in the pituitary gland or testicles), or a physical issue such as a blockage in the sperm duct.

Prostate Health

Although it's often involved in urinary problems in men, the prostate is technically part of the reproductive system (it makes semen, the fluid that carries sperm). The prostate is a walnut-sized gland that sits on top of the urethra, which is the tube that carries urine from the bladder. It naturally gets larger as a man ages, but if it gets too big it can cause urinary complications and other problems.

There are three types of problems that can occur in the prostate. The first is inflammation or infection, also known as prostatitis, which is usually indicated by a burning sensation while urinating. The second is prostate enlargement, or *benign prostatic hyperplasia* (BPH), which is a noncancerous enlargement of the gland generally accompanied by the urge to urinate frequently, a weak urine stream, and dribbling of urine. Nocturia, or increased urination at night, is another symptom. BPH is the most common prostate problem for men over fifty. By the time they're sixty, over half of men have some prostate enlargement (that number goes to 90 percent by age seventy).

ALERT!

Benign prostatic hyperplasia, or BPH, can be more than an annoyance. Recent research shows that as many as one in four men admitted to a hospital with acute urinary retention (AUR), which is a sudden inability to pass urine and is a common complication of advanced BPH, will die within a year.

The third type of prostate problem is cancer. Prostate cancer is the second most common type of cancer in American men, with 186,000 new cases and 29,000 deaths each year.

Conventional medicine treats BPH symptoms with drugs like finasteride (Proscar) and dutasteride (Avodart), which shrink the prostate gland by blocking the actions of testosterone. Other BPH drugs include alpha-adrenergic receptor blockers, which help relax the muscle of the prostate and bladder to relieve pressure and improve urine flow; they include doxazosin mesylate (Cardura) and tamsulosin hydrochloride (Flomax). Common side effects include dizziness, headache, and fatigue. Herbal alternatives include:

- **Nettle**
  (*Urtica dioica*)

  Nettle has been used for centuries in Europe to treat the symptoms of BPH. Modern studies suggest that it can slow the growth of prostate cells and blunt the BPH-related effects of testosterone.

- **Pumpkin**
  (*Cucurbita pepo*)

  Extracts of pumpkin seed oil, taken alone or combined with other herbs, can reduce BPH symptoms and shrink prostate tissues. Pumpkin contains a cholesterol-like substance called beta-sisterol, which seems to inhibit prostate enlargement; it's also found in soy (*Glycine max*).

- **Saw palmetto**
  (*Serenoa repens*)

  Several studies have shown that saw palmetto can relieve frequent and painful urination, urgency, and nocturia, and improve urinary flow. Its effects are similar to the drugs Flomax and Proscar—and it's better tolerated.

- **Pygeum**
  (*Prunus africana*)

  Numerous studies show that pygeum decreases nocturia, increases peak urine flow, and reduces residual urine volume.

- **Rye grass**
  (*Secale cereale*)

  Rye grass extracts have been shown to decrease frequency, nocturia, urgency, and prostate size, and increase urine flow.

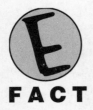

FACT

Conventional nondrug treatments for BPH include transurethral microwave thermotherapy, which uses a catheter to administer microwaves that destroy excess prostate tissue; water-induced thermotherapy, which accomplishes the same thing with hot water; and transurethral resection of the prostate, which is the most common type of BPH surgery.

Sleep Problems

Many men have problems with sleep: getting enough sleep, getting good quality sleep, and fighting sleepiness throughout the day.

Insomnia in men is most often tied to lifestyle factors like obesity, alcohol consumption, or physical inactivity, but it can also be the result of a psychiatric or medical problem such as joint or lower back pain, asthma, or acid reflux.

Conventional treatments for insomnia include sedating or sleep-inducing drugs—over-the-counter drugs like diphenhydramine HCI (Nytol, Sominex) and prescription meds like zolpidem tartrate (Ambien) and eszopiclone (Lunesta)—all of which carry the risk of side effects like dependence and "rebound insomnia" (when you stop taking the drug, your insomnia is worse than before).

Snoring and Sleep Apnea

Men—especially men who are overweight—often snore at night, which can be infuriating for their partners and can also cause health problems. Snoring reduces the quality of your sleep and can leave you feeling chronically tired, cranky, or mentally fuzzy.

Some snorers develop a condition called *obstructive sleep apnea*, or OSA, which is caused by a blockage in an upper airway. OSA involves loud, irregular snoring, which is broken up by repeated episodes of interrupted breathing—from ten to thirty seconds each. These episodes cause the body to release hormones that interrupt sleep, usually not so much that you regain consciousness but enough to leave you exhausted in the morning.

In many cases, OSA is tied to allergies, which can be treated with herbs such as flax (*Linum usitatissimum*) and evening primrose (*Oenothera biennis*) oils (see Chapter 9). Apnea that's tied to obesity can also be treated herbally (see Chapter 16).

Conventional medicine generally treats OSA with continuous positive airway pressure (CPAP), which is administered via a mask and machine that blows air into your mouth and nose at night to keep your airways open.

Some doctors also prescribe stimulant drugs like modafinil (Provigil) and armodafinil (Nuvigil), which can combat the daytime sleepiness associated with OSA but can also produce side effects such as anxiety, dizziness, headache, loss of muscle strength, and tingly or prickly sensations.

Herbal Answers

Herbal remedies for sleep problems include:

- **Kava**
  (*Piper methysticum*)

  Research shows that this herb can be as effective as the drug Valium in creating the changes in brain waves that help you fall—and stay—asleep.

- **Lemon balm**
  (*Melissa officinalis*)

  Studies show this mildly sedating herb can help relieve stress-related sleeplessness.

- **Valerian**
  (*Valeriana officinalis*)

  Centuries of use (and modern research) show that valerian can shorten the time it takes to fall asleep (sleep latency) and improve sleep quality.

CHAPTER 5

Older Adults

In the United States today, the number of seniors—and their percentage of the entire population—is at a record high and getting higher. According to the latest government statistics, there are now more than 35 million people over the age of sixty-five in the United States (that's 12 percent of the population). By 2030, a full 20 percent—more than 71 million people—will be sixty-five or older.

Living Longer—and Better?

Life expectancy in the U.S. continues to increase—men can expect to live to seventy-five years, and women to eighty. At the same time, mortality from diseases like cancer and cardiovascular disease are declining, meaning more and more Americans are surviving—and thriving—in their Golden Years.

Studies show that it's never too late to improve your health. Seniors can see big benefits from fairly small changes, reducing obesity, cancer, osteoporosis, and cardiovascular disease by as much as 50 percent simply by improving their diet and exercise habits. In some cases, seniors reap more health benefits from these lifestyle changes than any other age group.

But despite the drop in rates of deadly diseases, chronic conditions like high blood pressure (hypertension) and osteoarthritis continue to plague seniors. Chronic diseases are the leading cause of death in older Americans and are also responsible for roughly two-thirds of all health care costs (and 95 percent of seniors' health care expenditures). According to the Centers for Disease Control and Prevention (CDC), more than 80 percent of American seniors are living with at least one chronic condition, and 50 percent have at least two.

ESSENTIAL

In the absence of disease, aging is a fairly noneventful process, and many people can maintain their regular activities for many years after retirement. Getting older doesn't necessarily mean losing your health. In fact, many of the things that were once thought of as "normal" signs of aging, like wrinkles, cataracts, and arthritis, are now known to be signs of a disease process (or evidence of exposure to environmental factors that can be avoided).

The most common chronic conditions—including hypertension, arthritis, heart disease, diabetes, and stroke—cause pain, disability, and loss of functioning (and independence) for millions of people, and many produce cumulative and potentially fatal damage if left untreated.

Herbal medicine is uniquely suited to treating and preventing many of the chronic conditions that affect seniors. That's because herbs work gently—and synergistically—within the body instead of attacking a single problem or masking symptoms. They work with your body's own processes, not against them, meaning they support your body's efforts to maintain health and help your body defend itself against a disease instead of attacking the disease itself.

Seniors and Health

Seniors have a unique set of health concerns. Their bodies are different from anyone else's, they're prone to different diseases and conditions, and in many cases their attitudes toward health care are different, too.

Aging produces changes in body weight and composition—both men and women typically get heavier as they enter the senior ranks, then tend to lose weight as they move into their seventies. As you get older, your body also becomes less efficient at regulating blood pressure, body temperature, and the balance of fluids.

Some diseases that are common in older people can disrupt cell production. For example, Alzheimer's disease can cause the premature death of brain cells, and Parkinson's disease can kill off too many nerve cells. In contrast, cancer slows normal cell death and allows cancer cells to multiply and spread instead of dying off like they're supposed to. All of these changes affect how you live—how much and what kind of exercise you do, for example—as well as your health care needs.

Like any other segment of the population, seniors have a specific set of concerns regarding health care. But not all seniors are the same. No two people age at the same rate, and even within one person, not all body systems change in perfect harmony.

Seniors typically metabolize medicines, whether herbal or pharmaceutical, differently than younger people.

For example, because seniors typically weigh less and have a greater percentage of body fat, they have less lean muscle. As the ratio of body fat increases, the body reacts differently to drugs and other substances that are metabolized in fatty tissue, meaning that these substances typically remain in the body longer and thus may have stronger effects. Other substances accumulate because kidney function declines as people age. Nonsteroidal anti-inflammatory drugs, or NSAIDs, are more likely to cause gastrointestinal bleeding and kidney problems in seniors.

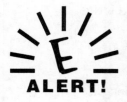

ALERT!

Many pharmaceuticals used by seniors can interact with herbs. For example, blood thinners and anticlotting agents can interact with Asian ginseng (*Panax ginseng*), dong quai (*Angelica sinensis*), ginkgo (*Ginkgo biloba*), ginger (*Zingiber officinale*), feverfew (*Tanacetum parthenium*), and garlic (*Allium sativum*). Heart medications like digoxin (Lanoxin) can cause problems when combined with Asian ginseng or Saint John's wort (*Hypericum perforatum*).

All of this means that seniors should follow herbal dosing directions carefully. Most experts recommend people over seventy should take about 80 percent of the recommended adult dose of any herbal remedy; seniors who are very frail (or sensitive to other medications) should start at half the recommended dose. For more information on safety and possible interactions, see Chapter 17.

Cardiovascular Concerns

As you age, your heart muscle becomes less efficient and has to work harder to keep the blood circulating throughout your body. Blood vessels also suffer with age, becoming less elastic. As a result, cardiovascular disease, or CVD—a group of conditions that includes heart disease, hypertension, and stroke—becomes increasingly common in older people. For more information on CVD, see Chapter 7.

Burgeoning Blood Pressure

High blood pressure, a.k.a. hypertension, is a chronic condition involving elevated pressure of blood against the artery walls. It affects more than 65 million Americans, or one in three adults, and is most common in seniors (nearly 71 percent of adults over sixty-five have been diagnosed).

Chronic hypertension can leave your heart enlarged, which can cause heart failure. And it can create aneurysms, or bulges, in your arteries and other blood vessels, which can cause sudden death. Hypertension also can lead to atherosclerosis (see below), kidney failure, and blindness, and is the single biggest risk factor for stroke.

ALERT!

Cholesterol is tied to more than diet and family history. Several disorders that are common in seniors, including diabetes and hypothyroidism (low thyroid gland activity), can raise your cholesterol levels. And some prescription drugs, including steroidal anti-inflammatories like prednisone, dexamethasone, and hydrocortisone, can also affect lipid levels.

Hyperlipidemia, or High Cholesterol

Many seniors have *hyperlipidemia*, or elevated blood lipids (including cholesterol), which is one of the biggest risk factors for heart attack and stroke. Cholesterol is a soft, waxy substance that occurs throughout the body. Some is produced by the liver, some comes from food (especially eggs and meat). Cholesterol comprises a few different lipids: low-density lipoprotein (LDL), known as "bad cholesterol" because it tends to remain in the body, where it oxidizes and accumulates in your arteries as plaque, and high-density lipoprotein (HDL), the "good" cholesterol that's generally eliminated from the body. Triglycerides are another type of lipid that's measured along with LDL and HDL and included in your total cholesterol. Ideally, you'll keep your total cholesterol (and LDL and triglycerides) low and your HDL high.

Hardening (and Clogged) Arteries

Arteriosclerosis is a general term for the thickening and hardening of arteries that occurs naturally as you get older. *Atherosclerosis*, which is a type of arteriosclerosis, involves the buildup of plaque, which is made up of cholesterol, cellular waste products, and other things that can accumulate in your arteries, narrowing and stiffening the passages.

Treatment Options

Conventional medicine treats CVD with drugs called ACE inhibitors, calcium channel blockers, and beta blockers, which can cause headaches, dizziness, fatigue, and nausea. Hyperlipidemia is generally treated with statin drugs, which decrease production of cholesterol by the liver and include atorvastatin (Lipitor) and rosuvastatin (Crestor); other drugs inhibit the absorption of dietary cholesterol, and include ezetimibe (Zetia), which recently was proven ineffective in preventing heart disease. These medicines can cause abdominal, back, and joint pain, among other things.

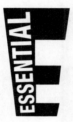

Purple grape (*Vitis vinifera*) juice, along with red wine, can lower blood pressure. Research shows that the chemicals in grapes work like a natural ACE inhibitor in the body (they decrease levels of angiotensin-converting enzyme, which constricts blood vessels in and around the heart).

But there are alternatives, including:

- **Alfalfa** (*Medicago sativa*)

  The aboveground parts of this nutrient-rich plant can lower serum cholesterol levels.

- **Artichoke** (*Cynara cardunculus, C. scolymus*)

  Extracts of this Mediterranean thistle lower cholesterol in a few ways. They stimulate the liver to release more bile, which helps eliminate dietary cholesterol and fat. And, like statin drugs, they inhibit a cholesterol-generating enzyme, so your body can't make as much of its own. Artichoke extract also seems to improve your HDL/LDL ratio, and its antioxidants prevent LDL from turning into plaque.

- **Flax** (*Linum usitatissimum*)

  High-fiber flaxseeds attach to cholesterol and prevent it from being absorbed. Research shows that taking almost any kind of flax—whole seeds, ground seeds, even muffins made with flax—can lower your cholesterol.

- **Guggul** (*Commiphora wightii, C. mukul*)

  Ayurvedic practitioners use the resin from the guggul tree to treat hyperlipidemia. Studies have shown that guggul extracts can lower total cholesterol, "bad" cholesterol, and triglycerides.

- **Maritime pine**
  (*Pinus pinaster*)

  Pine bark extracts can reduce blood pressure in cases of mild hypertension.

- **Olive**
  (*Olea europaea*)

  There's evidence that replacing other dietary fats with olive oil can lower your cholesterol and significantly reduce your risk of heart attack. Adding onion (*Allium cepa*) to your diet could also help lower your lipids.

- **Pomegranate**
  (*Punica granatum*)

  Research shows that this antioxidant-rich fruit can improve several markers of CVD, including atherosclerosis, hypertension, ischemia (restricted blood flow), and elevated cholesterol.

- **Turmeric**
  (*Curcuma longa*)

  Studies show that this anti-inflammatory and antioxidant spice can counteract high blood pressure and prevent heart failure.

- **Garlic**
  (*Allium sativum*)

  Garlic has been shown to decrease the oxidation of LDL cholesterol, which is the mechanism that damages the heart arteries.

Maintaining Your Vision

Getting older also affects your eyes. They begin to produce fewer tears and also undergo structural changes: The retinas get thinner, the lenses get cloudier, and the irises lose flexibility, all of which mean loss in eyesight. In addition, seniors with diabetes are at risk of diabetic retinopathy, which can also cause vision problems.

Cataracts

A cataract is a clouding of the eye's lens. It doesn't hurt, but it can interfere with your vision and make it harder to read or drive a car. Age is the biggest risk factor for cataracts: About half of Americans over the age of sixty-five have some degree of cataract formation, and by the age of seventy-five, about 70 percent have cataracts serious enough to interfere with their vision.

Other factors that can contribute to cataracts include diabetes, excessive sun exposure, smoking, and prolonged use of corticosteroid medications.

Glaucoma

Glaucoma, a leading cause of vision loss and blindness in the United States, is actually a group of diseases that create excessive pressure inside the eye and damage the optic nerve, which takes the images that your retina picks up and transfers them to your brain. Glaucoma can reduce your peripheral vision or create "blind spots." If left untreated, it can cause total blindness.

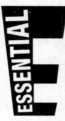

> To save your sight, most experts recommend upping your dietary intake of plant foods such as leafy green vegetables and brightly colored fruits, which contain antioxidants such as vitamins C and E, beta-carotene, riboflavin, lutein, and lycopene. There's extensive research that these nutrients can stave off age-related eye problems.

As with cataracts, age is the biggest risk factor (anyone over sixty is considered at risk). Glaucoma strikes blacks and Hispanics more often than whites, and is also more common in people who are nearsighted. Other risk factors include diabetes and corticosteroid use.

Macular Degeneration

Age-related macular degeneration, or AMD, is the leading cause of blindness and serious vision loss in seniors and affects more than 10 million Americans. AMD involves deterioration of the macula, which are cells shaped like cones and rods in your retina that control your ability to see what's in the center of your field of vision.

Age is the biggest factor in developing AMD, but it's also more common in women and whites (especially people with light-colored eyes). Cardiovascular disease, smoking, obesity, and long-term exposure to sunlight can also up your risk.

Diabetic Retinopathy

As its name implies, this is a disease of the retina that often accompanies diabetes—in fact, as many as 45 percent of diabetics have some degree of retinopathy. It's caused by diabetes-induced damage to the blood vessels in the retina and can create symptoms ranging from mild vision problems to total blindness. It's one of the biggest causes of blindness in U.S. adults. For more on diabetes, see Chapter 7.

Treatments for Eye Troubles

Because these conditions can advance rapidly and cause serious consequences, you should see your doctor immediately if you experience any significant changes in your vision. Advanced cases of eye disease may require surgery or other procedures (macular degeneration is sometimes treated with a laser).

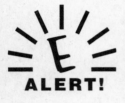

Consuming lots of omega-3 fatty acids—the essential fatty acids (EFAs) found in flax (*Linum usitatissimum*) seeds and oil—has been associated with lower rates of age-related macular degeneration. Flax is one of the few nonanimal sources of omega-3s (they're mostly found in fatty fish like salmon).

Anti-inflammatory drugs, including steroids, are also prescribed in some cases. Several herbs have been proven effective in preventing eye diseases and lessening their progression and symptoms. They include:

- **Bilberry** (*Vaccinium myrtillus*) — Bilberry and its cousin the blueberry (*Vaccinium angustifolium*) contain a number of antioxidants. They've been proven effective against several age-related eye disorders, including cataracts, macular degeneration, and retinopathy caused by diabetes and hypertension.

- **Ginkgo** (*Ginkgo biloba*) — Ginkgo has proven antioxidant effects and has been shown to improve vision in people with diabetic retinopathy, glaucoma, and AMD.

- **Grape** (*Vitis vinifera*) — Grape seeds contain powerful antioxidants called proanthocyanidins, which reduce oxidative damage to eye tissues. Research shows that grape seed extracts can improve vision and decrease eye stress.

- **Maritime pine** (*Pinus pinaster*) — Taking pine bark extracts can halt the progression of diabetic and other types of retinopathy and improve vision.

Healthy Bones and Joints

Getting older means losing bone mass and density: Bones are at their peak in your early thirties and go downhill from there. This creates changes, some harmless (you might get shorter) and some problematic (you can develop osteoporosis and be more prone to fractures). Many seniors also develop osteoarthritis from years of wear and tear on their joints.

The Challenges of Osteoarthritis

Osteoarthritis is a chronic condition that attacks the cartilage in the joints, wearing it away and eventually leaving bone rubbing against bone. Osteoarthritis is the most common type of arthritis, in seniors as well as the rest of the population. See Chapter 8 for more.

Osteoporosis

Osteoporosis involves a loss of bone mineral density that can lead to fractures. It occurs most often—about 80 percent of the time—in postmenopausal women, but it can also strike men or people with hormonal imbalances or who have used steroidal medications.

Around age thirty, most people stop building more bone, and the process of degradation begins. In women, this process accelerates right after menopause, but by age seventy, the rate of loss levels off in both men and women.

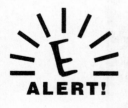

ALERT!

Many seniors can have balance and vision difficulties, suffer from conditions like Parkinson's disease and arthritis (which can affect gait), and take one or more medications—including antidepressants and antianxiety drugs that can cause muscular problems, dizziness, and confusion—all of which make them vulnerable to falls.

Falls and Fractures

According to the CDC, one of every three U.S. seniors falls each year. Fractures are the most serious consequence of falling, and bones that are weaker than average due to osteoporosis simply break more easily. In fact, half of all women and a quarter of all men will have an osteoporosis-related fracture in their lifetimes.

Treatment Options

Conventional medicine treats osteoarthritis with NSAIDs, which can cause stomach bleeding and increased risk of heart attack. Many people also use topical creams that contain capsaicin, which is the primary constituent of the herb cayenne (*Capsicum annuum, C. frutescens*). Osteoporosis is usually treated with a class of drugs called bisphosphonates, the best known of which is alendronate (Fosamax). Fosamax can cause abdominal pain, gas, acid reflux, bone and joint pain, and nausea. Herbal treatments for osteoporosis include:

- **Evening primrose oil** (*Oenothera biennis*)

  The seeds of this plant are rich in gamma-linolenic acid (GLA) and linoleic acid, which are used in the body to manufacture anti-inflammatory substances. Studies show that taking evening primrose oil can decrease bone turnover and increase bone mineral density in people with osteoporosis.

- **Red clover** (*Trifolium pratense*)

  The isoflavones in red clover seem to inhibit bone loss in women by acting like weak estrogens in the body.

- **Soy** (*Glycine max*)

  Soy can both prevent bone loss and increase bone mineral density. Research has shown that soy can reduce signs of osteoporosis in pre- and postmenopausal women.

- **Tea** (*Camellia sinensis*)

  Tea contains compounds that seem to build and strengthen bone. Research suggests that drinking green tea for several years can increase bone mineral density in both men and women.

Herbs for osteoarthritis include the following:

- **Devil's claw** (*Harpagophytum procumbens*)

  Studies show that extracts of this South African herb can reduce osteoarthritis pain.

- **Ginger**
  (*Zingiber officinale*)

  Ginger is an anti-inflammatory, and studies have shown that ginger extracts can reduce the pain of osteoarthritis. Ginger also seems to act as a structure-modifying agent, meaning it can foster changes in the arthritic joints instead of just masking the pain.

- **Guggul**
  (*Commiphora wightii,
  C. mukul*)

  This Indian shrub produces a resin that's a traditional Ayurvedic remedy for arthritis. Modern researchers have shown that oral preparations can relieve osteoarthritis pain.

- **Nettle**
  (*Urtica dioica*)

  Best known as an herbal remedy for allergies, nettle extracts—taken orally or applied topically—seem to reduce arthritis pain, too.

Keeping Your Mind Sharp

As you age, the number of neurons, or nerve cells, in your brain naturally decreases, and you may notice changes in your short-term memory and other cognitive functions. Everyone can expect to develop some degree of age-related cognitive impairment, but some seniors will also develop dementia, which is a more serious condition.

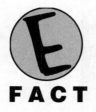

Research shows that maintaining an active social life can significantly reduce your risk of dementia and Alzheimer's disease. Older people who have large social networks—and maintain daily contact with friends and loved ones—are much less likely to develop dementia and more likely to maintain cognitive functioning.

Dementia

Dementia is not a disease, *per se*, but instead is a group of symptoms—including loss of memory, reasoning, planning, and social abilities—caused by degeneration of the tissues in the brain. It is diagnosed when a person shows impairment in two or more brain functions severe enough to interfere with daily functioning; it's not associated with a loss of alteration or consciousness (meaning it's not a type of amnesia) and it has not been present since birth (it's not a congenital condition).

Although most people with dementia are elderly, dementia is not an inevitable part of aging. It's caused by a group of brain diseases, of which Alzheimer's disease is the most common.

Mild Cognitive Impairment (MCI)

Mild cognitive impairment is a type of dementia that lies somewhere between the changes of normal aging and the serious deficits of Alzheimer's. While it's not a definite predictor of Alzheimer's, people with MCI are three to four times more likely to develop AD than people without it. Experts at the Mayo Clinic estimate that 12 percent of people over the age of seventy have MCI.

Alzheimer's Disease

Alzheimer's disease (AD), the most common cause of dementia in older people, affects about 5 million Americans—roughly 5 percent of people between sixty-five to seventy-four and nearly half of those over the age of eighty-five.

Treatment Options

There is no cure for dementia. Treatments—both conventional and herbal—focus on improving the patient's quality of life and delaying, as much as possible, the disease's progression.

AD drugs include galantamine (Razadyne) and donepezil (Aricept), which boost the levels of an enzyme called *choline acetyltransferase* that's in short supply in people with Alzheimer's. These drugs can produce side effects like diarrhea, fatigue, insomnia, muscle cramps, nausea, and vomiting.

Several herbs have a long history of use as brain aids, and several have shown promise against age-related cognitive decline, dementia, and Alzheimer's, and can be taken in conjunction with conventional AD remedies.

• **Garlic** (*Allium sativum*)	Aged extracts of garlic have been proven in numerous studies to reduce inflammation and cholesterol levels, which can contribute to the development of dementia.

- **Ginkgo**
  (*Ginkgo biloba*)

  The best known of the cognition-boosting botanicals, ginkgo has proven antioxidant and anti-inflammatory actions and has been shown to fight normal age-related cognitive decline as well as cerebral insufficiency (impaired blood flow to the brain) and several types of clinical dementia. Ginkgo has been shown to improve memory and attention in healthy young people, too.

- **Grape**
  (*Vitis vinifera*)

  Several studies have found that drinking red wine is associated with lower incidence of Alzheimer's disease. Other research has shown that extracts of grape seeds and skin can reduce age-related dementia and cognitive loss.

- **Lemon balm**
  (*Melissa officinalis*)

  Extracts of this herb, long revered for its ability to calm anxiety, have been shown to reduce symptoms of mild to moderate Alzheimer's disease.

- **Rooibos**
  (*Aspalathus linearis*)

  Research shows that this South African "tea" can offset the damage to the central nervous system caused by aging.

- **Sage**
  (*Salvia officinalis,*
  S. lavandulaefolia)

  Sage extracts have been shown to improve cognitive function in people with mild to moderate Alzheimer's. Sage can also improve memory in younger people.

- **Turmeric**
  (*Curcuma longa*)

  This aromatic South Asian spice contains a chemical called curcumin, which has been shown to inhibit the oxidation and other processes that are behind AD and other neurodegenerative diseases.

CHAPTER 6

Caring for Kids

Having children today almost always means having a medicine cabinet that's jammed with bottles of brightly colored syrups and tablets, all promising to obliterate a child's sniffles or tummy ache before bedtime. But most common childhood illnesses are mild—you've got to control the symptoms and help your child feel better, not eradicate a million life-threatening microbes—so many drug treatments are overkill. Herbs work to gently ease your child's discomfort and help his body heal itself.

Children and Herbal Remedies

Most childhood illnesses—diaper rash, ear and upper respiratory infections—are fairly mild, requiring more symptom management than serious medical intervention. Most often, you'll want to keep your child comfortable and, when necessary, bolster his natural immunity to get him back on the playground as soon as possible.

Because it's focused so heavily on prevention and the fostering of overall good health, herbal medicine is uniquely suited to treat most of the common ills of childhood. Compare that to conventional medicine, which focuses on the elimination of specific symptoms or pathogens, and you'll see that, in many cases, conventional medicine overmedicates children and may actually encourage future health problems.

Consider atopic dermatitis, which is an allergic skin condition common in babies and children. Conventional medicine uses steroidal or immune-modulating medications, which work well in the short term but might turn a childhood case of itchy skin into a lifelong problem.

Of course, there are times when the powerful drugs of Western medicine are required. But there are also plenty of times that call for the gentler healing of herbs.

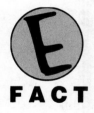

FACT

Modern pharmaceuticals are extremely effective at relieving many childhood illnesses, but most prescription and over-the-counter drugs produce unwanted side effects and may even make your child sicker. For example, decongestants can actually create recurring (or "rebound") congestion, while antibiotics have been linked to the development of drug-resistant superbugs.

Common Kids' Concerns

Children are not small adults, and their needs can be quite different from grownups'. Children have more skin (surface area) per pound than adults do, meaning remedies applied topically can have a stronger effect. Kids' bodies also have a different internal composition (the ratio of fat to water), and the organs that metabolize drugs, including the liver, don't function the same way. Young children also have a less well-developed blood-brain barrier, meaning more drugs or other agents can reach the central nervous system with potentially toxic results. Here are a few steps to take before using any herbal remedies on your child:

- **Talk to your pediatrician.** Be sure to discuss any therapies—including herbs—you're considering. If your child has specific concerns, be sure you've got a confirmed diagnosis before proceeding with herbal remedies.
- **Get professional help.** If you're treating a serious condition, consider working with a trained herbalist or natural medicine practitioner (see Chapter 18).
- **Don't guess on the dosage.** As with adults, you should keep in mind this rule: More isn't always better. For advice on dosages, see Chapter 18.

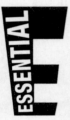

Herbal remedies can be very effective in children, but some have a strong or unpleasant flavor that kids won't like (especially kids who are used to taking artificially flavored cough syrups and other "children's" medicines). Try mixing an unpalatable remedy with some honey or applesauce to mask the taste.

Although the majority of herbal preparations are well tolerated by children, you should understand the actions and potential side effects of any herb you're giving to your child. Here are some rules to remember when treating children with herbs:

- **Don't give medicine of any kind**—including herbal—to a baby younger than six months (speak with your pediatrician before treating an infant's health issues at home).
- **When using herbal treatments on your child,** be sure to allow a few weeks before you decide that a remedy is or isn't working. If your

child has a bad reaction to anything, discontinue using it. Speak with your pediatrician if the reaction is serious.

- **Watch your child for any indication**—good or bad—that the herb is having an effect. If your child shows signs of sensitivity, such as headache, rash, or upset stomach, stop using it.
- **Treat herbs as you would any medications:** Keep them out of reach of your children (and pets), and store in a cool, dry place unless otherwise instructed.
- **Don't treat a high fever** (over 101°Fahrenheit in infants, 102°F in toddlers, or 103°F in older children) at home. Likewise, if your child has a stiff neck or headache along with a fever, or if she develops an ear infection that doesn't clear up within twenty-four hours, get immediate medical attention.

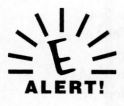

ALERT!

Avoid giving your child any herb that's a stimulant, such as guarana (*Paullinia cupana*). You should also avoid herbs with laxative properties, like cascara sagrada (*Frangula purshiana*) and senna (*Cassia officinalis, Senna alexandrina*), and herbs with hormonal effects, such as black cohosh (*Actaea racemosa, Cimicifuga racemosa*) or red clover (*Trifolium pratense*).

Bringing Up Baby

Babies arrive with a unique set of health issues, many of which they'll grow out of by their first birthday. But in that first year, you'll probably have to deal with several issues, from teething to tummy troubles.

Teething

Teething is the process by which a baby gets her first set of teeth—they grow out of the gums on her upper and lower jaws, breaking through the skin on the way (and causing the gums to redden and swell and the baby to drool and chew on anything she can get into her mouth). Teething should never be accompanied by a fever; see your doctor if your baby is running a fever.

Some pediatricians recommend topical analgesics like benzocaine or oral pain relievers like acetaminophen; aspirin should never be given to children younger than eighteen because it increases the risk of getting Reye's syndrome, a potentially life-threatening condition. Herbal options for teething include:

- **Chamomile** (*Matricaria recutita*)
  An infusion of chamomile works as a safe, gentle pain reliever and a very mild sedative—perfect for soothing fussy babies. It can also help heal inflamed tissues.

- **Slippery elm** (*Ulmus rubra*)
  Slippery elm has demulcent properties, meaning it can be soothing to sore gums when applied topically.

Colic

All babies cry, but colicky babies cry more—and with more gusto. Colic is unexplained, persistent crying in healthy babies and affects as many as 25 percent of children. It's defined as crying that goes on for more than three hours a day, at least three days a week, and persists for more than three weeks. A baby with colic typically clenches his fists, curls his legs, or otherwise acts as if he's in pain, screaming and often turning bright red in the process. Colicky babies can also have a distended belly that feels hard to the touch.

In most cases, colic clears up by the time the baby is six months old. If your baby is still colicky after that—or if he shows symptoms of illness, such as vomiting, fever, or diarrhea—see your pediatrician.

Some conventional medical practitioners recommend simethicone (Mylicon), an over-the-counter (OTC) pain reliever and antigas medicine, which can cause diarrhea. Here are some herbal alternatives for colic:

- **Chamomile** (*Matricaria recutita*)
  Chamomile can relieve intestinal spasms and reduce inflammation in gastrointestinal tissues. In one study, infants given a multiherb tea containing chamomile showed significantly improved colic symptoms.

- **Fennel** (*Foeniculum vulgare*)
  Fennel seed oil is a traditional colic remedy. Modern research has shown that it can eliminate colic symptoms without side effects.

- **Lavender** (*Lavandula angustifolia*)
  Lavender essential oil is known to relax both body and mind—and a bath or massage that incorporates it can help a colicky baby get some sleep.

Children's Skin Conditions

Babies and toddlers can develop a few unique skin problems that require special, extra-gentle care.

Diaper Rash

The bane of many a baby's bottom, diaper rash is most often caused by contact with soiled diapers (or a reaction to baby wipes or laundry detergent). It's a very common condition that can leave a baby's skin red, scaly, and very tender.

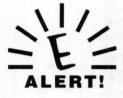

Talc, the key ingredient in baby powder, has been a classic in American nurseries for generations. But talcum powder has been linked to respiratory problems and even cancer. Safer stand-ins: dried and powdered formulations of the herbs arrowroot (*Maranta arundinacea*) or rice (*Oryza sativa*), or the dried, starchy component of corn (*Zea mays*).

A case of diaper rash that lasts for more than three days and includes areas of raised red bumps and a series of small red patches extending out beyond the main rash could be the sign of an infection with *Candida albicans*, a yeast-like fungus.

Dermatitis

Babies are prone to a few types of *dermatitis* (skin inflammation). Infantile seborrheic dermatitis, or cradle cap, is a nonallergic condition that produces thick, scaly patches on a baby's scalp. (In adults, it's called dandruff.) It's triggered by hormones passed from the mother, which cause the baby's scalp to produce too much sebum (oil), and usually clears on its own.

Atopic dermatitis, or infant eczema, appears at six to twelve weeks as a rash or patch of small pimples on the cheeks or chest and sometimes the elbows and knees.

Treatment Options

Conventional remedies for diaper rash include topical zinc oxide or petroleum jelly, which can cause allergic reactions. *Candida* infections might be treated with antifungals like clotrimazole (Mycelex) or nystatin (Mycostatin), which can cause skin reactions in some people.

Doctors generally advise parents to leave a case of cradle cap alone. Infant eczema is typically treated with hydrocortisone creams and ointments, which control itching but can cause skin reactions as more serious side effects if used long term or applied excessively.

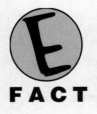

FACT

Eczema is caused by an immune system reaction that isn't fully understood. It can appear in infancy and then disappear. Or, it can recur throughout childhood and into adulthood (in some people, it doesn't appear until age four or five; in others, it starts in the adult years). In most babies, eczema resolves itself by age two.

Herbal alternatives include these:

- **Calendula** (*Calendula officinalis*)

  Calendula is an anti-inflammatory that can soothe and heal many rashes.

- **Lavender** (*Lavandula angustifolia*)

  This is a classic remedy for all kinds of skin inflammation, including diaper rash. New research shows that it's also effective against *Candida albicans*.

- **Rice bran** (*Oryza sativa*)

  Rice—or more specifically, its outer husk, or bran—has been used topically to treat a variety of inflammatory skin problems. Research has shown that adding a decoction of rice bran to a child's bath can relieve atopic dermatitis. Oats (*Avena sativa*) are also effective in anti-itch baths.

Tips for Toddlers

Toddlers—children who may still be "toddling" instead of walking perfectly —fall into the second stage of childhood development: not babies anymore, not yet schoolkids. Between the ages of one and three, toddlers are exploring their world and encountering new health challenges along the way.

Ear Infections

Infections of the middle chamber of the ear are called *otitis media (OM)*. In otitis media, the natural fluids within the ear don't drain properly, creating inflammation and pain.

Conventional medicine treats OM with pain-relieving drugs and, in many cases, antibiotics such as amoxicillin. But giving kids too many antibiotics can lead to recurrent infections and antibiotic resistance. Research suggests that as many as half of the children who are given antibiotics for recurrent otitis media will still have drug-resistant *pneumococcus* and other common OM bugs in their bodies.

If you think your child has an ear infection coming on, you might be able to stop it before it requires antibiotics. If an infection is already established, you can use these remedies in conjunction with antibiotics to reduce pain and speed healing.

• **Garlic** (*Allium sativum*)	Garlic is a proven antimicrobial that can be used topically (as oil-based drops) to treat otitis media in young children.
• **Goldenseal** (*Hydrastis canadensis*)	This is a classic herbal remedy that can be used internally and externally to fight ear infections. Its most beneficial constituent (at least as far as humans are concerned) is berberine, a potent antibacterial that seems to prevent germs from attaching themselves to cell membranes.
• **Lavender** (*Lavandula angustifolia*)	A natural anesthetic and anti-inflammatory, lavender oil, applied in a compress, can relieve the pain of an ear infection.
• **Saint John's wort** (*Hypericum perforatum*)	This herb is an antibacterial and anti-inflammatory. A recent study found that ear drops containing Saint John's wort and calendula (*Calendula officinalis*) were better than a pharmaceutical anesthetic at relieving OM pain.

Tummy Troubles

Stomachaches can be caused by many things, including infection (like gastroenteritis, or "stomach flu"), constipation, or a reaction to certain foods. Stress can also contribute.

Although most gastrointestinal (GI) problems in children resolve themselves, conventional doctors may recommend pharmaceuticals like bismuth subsalicylate (Pepto-Bismol), which can cause allergic reactions in some children and can also interact with other medications. Herbal alternatives include these:

- **Fennel** (*Foeniculum vulgare*)
Fennel is a natural anti-inflammatory, anesthetic, and analgesic, so it helps relieve stomach pain. It's also a natural antacid, meaning it can neutralize excess stomach acids.

- **Ginger** (*Zingiber officinale*)
This ancient remedy is gentle and safe for use in children. Research has demonstrated its effects as an antiemetic (it combats nausea and vomiting) and gastric stimulant (it speeds the movement of food through the GI tract).

- **Peppermint** (*Mentha x piperita*)
Peppermint is a traditional remedy for all sorts of GI problems, including diarrhea, indigestion, nausea, and vomiting. The oil contains menthol, which relaxes smooth muscles in the stomach and small intestine (and gives peppermint its kid-pleasing flavor).

- **Psyllium** (*Plantago ovata, P. psyllium*)
This high-fiber plant works as a gentle bulk-forming laxative.

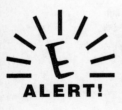

ALERT!

If your child is vomiting a lot or is in significant pain, or if you suspect that she has food poisoning or a food sensitivity, contact your pediatrician. Most cases of gastrointestinal distress in kids go away on their own, but vomiting, diarrhea, or other problems could be signs of a more serious problem.

Emotional and Behavioral Problems

Growing up means facing new social and developmental challenges, which can create anxiety and bring issues like attention difficulties to center stage.

Anxiety and Excitability

Most young children are lively, but excessive energy can be hard on both parent and child. Children who aren't emotionally mature enough to calm themselves get overly agitated, which can interfere with sleep as well as daytime functioning. Some young children also become anxious.

Parents looking for a way to safely calm a child—without pharmaceutical sedatives—should investigate the following herbs:

- **Chamomile** (*Matricaria recutita*)   This soothing herb can brew a mild, pleasant-tasting tea that can calm an agitated toddler. It also works in a bath.

- **Lemon balm** (*Melissa officinalis*)   Lemon balm is another gentle, kid-friendly remedy for anxiety. Recent research found that a combination of lemon balm and valerian (*Valeriana officinalis*) reduced restlessness and improved sleep in young children.

- **Passionflower** (*Passiflora incarnata*)   This is a classic remedy for anxiety, nervousness and excitability, and insomnia.

Attention Difficulties

Attention deficit hyperactivity disorder, or ADHD, is a behavioral disorder involving inattention, hyperactivity, and impulsivity that most often shows up in preschool or early elementary school; as many as 9 percent of American children aged eight to fifteen have symptoms.

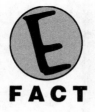

A recent study found that "green" outdoor activities—things that exposed kids to trees and grass—reduced ADHD symptoms significantly more than activities that were conducted in other (i.e., indoor) settings.

Conventional medicine most often treats ADHD with stimulants like amphetamines (Adderall) and methylphenidate hydrochloride (Ritalin) or atomoxetine hydrochloride (Strattera). Side effects can include decreased appetite, insomnia, anxiety, stomachache, or headache.

Herbalism offers a few alternatives (these herbs can also be used in conjunction with conventional ADHD treatments):

- **American ginseng**
  (*Panax quinquefolius*)

  Preliminary evidence has shown that a combination of ginkgo (*Ginkgo biloba*) and American ginseng extracts can reduce anxiety, hyperactivity, and impulsivity in children.

- **Flax**
  (*Linum usitatissimum*)

  Research shows that kids with ADHD have lower levels of omega-3 fatty acids, which are essential for psychological functioning. There's evidence that supplementing kids with omega-3s, like those in flax oil, can alleviate symptoms of ADHD.

- **Ginkgo**
  (*Ginkgo biloba*)

  It's best known for improving cognitive functioning in older people, but research shows that ginkgo can reduce anxiety, hyperactivity, and impulsivity in kids, too.

- **Maritime pine**
  (*Pinus pinaster*)

  An extract from this tree's bark has been shown to reduce hyperactivity and increase attentiveness and concentration in kids with ADHD.

Kids, Colds, and Flu

Most preschoolers and school-age kids get between six and ten colds every year (they don't call it the common cold for nothing). Influenza, a.k.a. "the flu," is much less common (and much more serious). It puts more than 20,000 children under the age of five into the hospital every year.

The flu can be especially tough on young children. Thus, the American Academy of Pediatrics (AAP) and the Centers for Disease Control and Prevention (CDC) recommend that all children between six months and five years old get a flu shot. For more on colds and flu, see Chapter 13. Several herbs can help keep a child's immunity high—and her risk of colds and flu low.

- **American ginseng**
  (*Panax quinquefolius*)

  American ginseng is an adaptogen—it increases the body's resistance to stress—and research shows it might decrease your child's risk of getting sick (and if he does, it can reduce the severity and duration of his symptoms).

- **Andrographis**
  (*Andrographis paniculata*)

  This herb seems to boost immune function. A combination of andrographis and eleuthero (*Eleutherococcus senticosus*) has been shown to significantly improve symptoms of the common cold in kids.

- **Echinacea**
  (*Echinacea purpurea*)

  Echinacea stimulates immunity and has been proven to reduce the severity and duration of colds.

- **Licorice**
  (*Glycyrrhiza glabra*)

  This is an ancient remedy for bronchial congestion, sore throat, and coughs—and most kids love the taste. It's a natural expectorant, cough-suppressant, and pain reliever.

- **Slippery elm**
  (*Ulmus rubra*)

  The "slippery" mucilage in this tree's inner bark makes a soothing remedy for cough-ravaged throats.

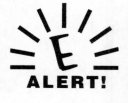

Cough and cold medicines can cause serious problems—and send about 7,000 kids to the hospital every year, most often because of accidental overdosing. Research shows that cold medicines seldom produce significant improvements in children, even when used properly, and they're not recommended at all for children under four.

Other Childhood Infections

By the time they reach kindergarten, most children are socially active (and thus exposed to plenty of disease-causing microbes), meaning very few kids can make it through a school year without at least one bout with a cold or other contagious disease.

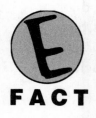

Chickenpox, an infection with a virus called *varicella zoster*, is one of the most common childhood diseases in the United States. However, it seems to be on its way out, thanks to a vaccine that was introduced in the mid-1990s. Chickenpox produces a series of small, itchy blisters that look like chickpeas (and give the disease its name), as well as fever and fatigue.

Infectious Diseases

Kids catch lots of infections that produce unpleasant symptoms, such as sore throat and cough (see above), as well as itching (as in chickenpox).

When your child gets an infection, unless she is running a high fever for more than a few days, you'll probably be advised to treat her at home, with OTC pain relievers (like acetaminophen) and calamine lotion for the itching. Herbal options include these:

- Calendula
  (*Calendula officinalis*)

  The flowers of the calendula, or garden marigold, plant contain anti-inflammatory and antibacterial agents, meaning calendula can relieve itching and help prevent the infection of any blisters that your child scratches.

- Oats
  (*Avena sativa*)

  Baths and topical preparations containing oats can relieve itching and irritation. Oats also help restore the skin's natural moisture barrier.

Head Lice

Kids aged three and up are likely to come home from day care, school, or summer camp with head lice (about one in every ten school-age kids gets them). An adult louse is about the size of a sesame seed, and its eggs, called *nits*, are even tinier (hence the term *nitpicking*).

Head lice are extremely contagious, and being in close, head-to-head contact with an infected person is the easiest way to get them. Head lice cause itching, and many children develop sores on their scalps from scratching. Conventional treatment for head lice involves louse-killing chemicals like prescription malathion (Ovide), which kills adult lice and some nits. It can cause scalp and eye irritation and is not intended for use on children younger than six. Another prescription option is benzene hexachloride/gamma-hexachlorocyclohexane (Lindane), a lotion or shampoo that kills lice and nits but can cause hair loss, headaches, and skin irritation.

The *Pediculus capitis* louse is becoming increasingly resistant to the chemical insecticides permethrin and pyrethroid, which are the active ingredients in most OTC head lice treatments. Lice in other parts of the world are showing resistance to malathion, which is sold as a prescription in the United States.

OTC remedies use pyrethrins or permethrins, both of which can cause skin reactions and respiratory problems. These drugs are not approved for use on children under two, and because they kill only adult or newly hatched lice, both require reapplication. Many herbs are toxic to lice—but not people—and include these:

- **Coconut**
  (*Cocos nucifera*)

  Coconut contains several insecticidal and larvicidal compounds. In one study, a combination of the essential oils of coconut and two other natural bug-killers, anise (*Pimpinella anisum*) and ylang-ylang (*Cananga odorata*), was as effective as the insecticides permethrin and malathion.

- **Eucalyptus**
  (*Eucalyptus globulus*)

  Eucalyptus oil contains several compounds that have been shown to be as effective as pharmaceuticals in killing lice and their eggs.

- **Neem**
  (*Azadirachta indica*)

  Research shows that neem-based shampoos and other treatments kill lice and nits with no irritation or other side effects.

- **Tea tree**
  (*Melaleuca alternifolia*)

  Tea tree oil contains a chemical called terpinol, which is lethal to lice. Combined with peppermint (*Mentha x. piperita*) and lavender (*Lavandula angustifolia*) oils, tea tree oil can also repel lice and discourage them from feeding.

The Grade School Years

Kids in grade school have their own set of health issues. Their bodies are changing and their social lives and activities are changing, too. Many kids in this age group are getting more active in sports, which brings a whole new set of health concerns.

Locker Room Woes

Children who participate in sports or gym class can develop a few types of fungal (or *tinea*) infections, including *tinea corporis* (also known as jock itch) and *tinea pedis* (better known as athlete's foot). These two very uncomfortable infections are caused by mold-like fungi knows as *dermatophytes*. These fungi are spread by direct contact (touching a hard surface or an infected person) and thrive in warm, wet environments like swimming pools and locker rooms.

Tinea infections are treated with OTC topical antifungals like terbinafine (Lamisil), which can cause reactions in some individuals. Herbal remedies can be used in place of these medicines, and include:

- **Clove**
  (*Syzygium aromaticum*)

  Clove oil contains high levels of eugenol, a potent antifungal; it also has several antiseptic and anti-inflammatory constituents. Research shows that clove and other plant oils can stop the proliferation of dermatophytes.

- **Echinacea**
  (*Echinacea purpurea*)

  This North American perennial herb can help your child fight almost any infection, including *tinea*. Echinacea can be used both internally and externally.

- **Lavender**
  (*Lavandula angustifolia*)

  A natural anesthetic and anti-inflammatory. It is also effective against many kinds of fungi.

- **Tea tree**
  (*Melaleuca alternifolia*)

  A traditional Aboriginal treatment for all types of skin inflammation and infections (including fungal), it can also speed healing of inflamed (or scratched-up) tissues.

Swimmer's Ear

Kids who spend a lot of time in the pool can get a type of infection known as swimmer's ear, or *otitis externa*. Swimmer's ear is an infection of the outer ear canal. It strikes when a child gets contaminated water into her ear, most often from a pool with poorly maintained chlorine or pH levels, or a lake that has high levels of bacteria. It's treated with OTC pain relievers and prescription antibiotics (see above). To kill bacteria preemptively, many conventional practitioners recommend treating the ears with hydrogen peroxide after every swim. Hydrogen peroxide can damage skin tissues and isn't a particularly effective antiseptic.

If your child complains of sore ears after swimming, you can try to clear it up with herbs before heading to the doctor for antibiotics. If she does need the drugs, you can use these remedies in conjunction with them:

- **Goldenseal**
  (*Hydrastis canadensis*)

  Can be taken internally or applied externally to help clear up an ear infection. Its astringent and antiseptic properties are especially helpful for waterlogged ears.

- **Saint John's wort**   Research shows that ear drops containing Saint John's wort can relieve
  (*Hypericum*   earache pain more quickly than pharmaceutical anesthetics.
  perforatum)

- **Witch hazel**   Witch hazel contains astringent, antiseptic, and antibacterial com-
  (*Hamamelis virginiana*) pounds, which makes it perfect for drying (and sanitizing) infected ears.

Teenagers

Once they're in high school, most kids are deep into the many social and health-related issues of being a teenager. They want to look good at all times, despite the many changes that are going on in their bodies.

Puberty and Pimples

Acne is the most common skin disorder in the United States and is especially problematic for the under-twenty set, thanks to rapidly shifting hormones. It's caused by excessive sebum production, which creates clogged pores and pimples that can become infected with *Propionibacterium acnes* bacteria. For more, see Chapter 15.

Conventional doctors recommend OTC treatments made with benzoyl peroxide, sulfur, and salicylic acid, which reduce pimples but can cause irritation and drying.

Prescription treatments include topical antibiotics and antibacterials and oral antibiotics; oral contraceptives are also prescribed for some female patients. Antibiotics can increase the likelihood of sunburn and affect a child's overall immunity. Birth control pills can cause digestive problems and headaches. Herbal acne remedies include these:

- **Calendula**   Calendula can soothe skin (it contains anti-inflammatory compounds)
  (*Calendula officinalis*) and also reduce *P. acnes* bacteria and oil (it has antibacterial and
                        astringent properties, too).

- **Guggul**   Used throughout India, guggul has antibacterial, anti-inflammatory,
  (*Commiphora wightii,* antiseptic, and immune-stimulating compounds. It's been proven as
  C. mukul)   effective as the prescription drug tetracycline against acne.

- **Tea tree**   Tea tree oil has antiseptic, antibacterial, and anti-inflammatory effects
  (*Melaleuca alternifolia*) and works as well as benzoyl peroxide—usually without side effects.

Body Odor

Puberty often means a big surge in perspiration, as sweat glands in the underarms become more active. Sweat by itself doesn't smell, but when it combines with bacteria it can produce body odor. Commercial deodorants kill bacteria and mask odor with chemical fragrance; antiperspirants inhibit the sweating process with aluminum salts (aluminum chloride, aluminum chlorohydrate, and aluminum zirconium). Most antiperspirants also contain fragrance.

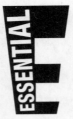

Chlorophyll, the chemical that makes green plants green, is a natural, works-from-the-inside deodorant. It's found in the greatest concentrations in dark-green plants like parsley (*Petroselinum crispum*) and spinach (*Spinacia oleracea*). Eating them (or other chlorophyll-rich herbs) or taking supplemental chlorophyllin, which is derived from chlorophyll, can reduce body odor and bad breath.

Aluminum compounds have been associated with serious health problems; aluminum itself is a known neurotoxin, and aluminum salts have demonstrated toxicity in laboratory animals. Fragrances used in cosmetics have been linked to a host of problems, including reproductive and developmental health risks. Natural options for perspiration and body odor include:

- **Camphor**
  (*Cinnamomum camphora*)

  The leaves of this plant contain a natural deodorant called terpinolene, plus fragrant (and antibacterial) oils, which make it an effective deodorant. Juniper (*Juniperus communis*) and rosemary (*Rosmarinus officinalis*) contain similar odor-fighting compounds.

- **Sage**
  (*Salvia officinalis,
  S. lavandulaefolia*)

  Sage is a classic remedy for excessive perspiration. It's also an antibacterial, meaning it can combat odor-causing bacteria, too.

- **Yarrow**
  (*Achillea millefolium*)

  A natural deodorant, yarrow also has astringent and antibacterial properties, making it perfect for drying up excess moisture and killing bacteria.

CHAPTER 7

Chronic Diseases and Conditions

Herbs have been used for centuries to treat all kinds of chronic disorders, including heart disease, stroke, diabetes, and cancer. And while conventional medicine has arguably made enormous strides against many chronic diseases, herbal medicine remains a valuable tool in both the prevention and treatment of many of these conditions.

The Problem of Chronic Disease

According to the Centers for Disease Control and Prevention (CDC), chronic diseases are the biggest causes of death and disability in this country. They account for 1.7 million deaths every year (that's 70 percent of all deaths) and cause major disabilities and lifestyle limitations for another 25 million Americans (almost 10 percent of the population).

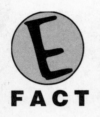

FACT

High-fat, calorie-dense foods and a sedentary existence are known causes of chronic disease. And as people in the developing world increasingly adopt this lifestyle, their rates of chronic disease are exploding. According to the World Health Organization, chronic disease, which now contributes to about 60 percent of deaths worldwide, will be responsible for nearly 75 percent by 2020.

Generally speaking, chronic diseases aren't preventable by any vaccine, nor can they be cured by medicines. They also don't just go away on their own. Most can be traced to either a genetic predisposition or a set of lifestyle factors—including the way you eat, exercise, and entertain yourself over the course of your life.

We know that many diseases and conditions, including heart disease, diabetes, obesity, cancer, alcoholism, and asthma, can run in families. Having a family member—especially a close relative—with a certain disease means you might have a higher chance of developing it than someone with no family history. But it doesn't mean that you'll definitely be affected. Genetics are only one part of the picture.

The biggest factor in most cases of chronic disease is health behavior: using (or avoiding) tobacco and alcohol, for example, or making healthy (or unhealthy) menu choices. Numerous studies have shown a clear connection between diet and chronic disease: Simply put, people who eat a plant-based diet, with more whole grains and lean protein and less red meat and processed foods, have less cancer, heart disease, diabetes, and obesity.

How Herbs Can Help

Chronic diseases are often associated with misguided processes within the body—normal and necessary operations that have gone awry and are creating complications that can set the stage for illness. And many herbs possess the exact constituents that are missing in someone with these problems.

A common denominator in many chronic diseases is *inflammation*, which is the body's natural reaction to an injury or invading pathogen and is a key component of the healing process. But prolonged or chronic inflammation leads to a cycle of destruction and healing that seems to perpetuate the development of disease by interfering with immune function.

For example, people with ulcerative colitis, a chronic inflammatory condition of the colon, are at a greater-than-average risk for colon cancer. And having a chronic inflammatory lung condition like asthma seems to increase your risk of lung cancer, even if you're not a smoker. Many herbs are natural anti-inflammatories, meaning they can help reduce the type of ongoing inflammation that's been associated with so many chronic diseases.

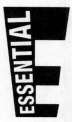

When it comes to chronic disease, small changes bring big results. For example, people who moderately reduced their blood pressure saw a 21 percent reduction in heart disease, a 37 percent drop in stroke, and a 13 percent reduction in overall mortality. Lowering your cholesterol by 10 percent can decrease your risk of heart disease by almost 30 percent.

Many chronic diseases are also associated with *oxidation*, which is a chemical reaction that occurs naturally throughout your body and in the outside world (it's what turns metal rusty and a slice of apple brown). Through oxidation, an oxidizing agent removes electrons from another substance; this reaction can produce molecules called *free radicals*, which can damage cells. In a healthy body, free radicals are kept in check by molecules called *antioxidants*. If there aren't enough antioxidants around, the cells can sustain oxidative damage, also known as oxidative stress, which is known to play a role in many chronic diseases.

Many herbs are powerful antioxidants, meaning they can blunt the damaging and disease-producing effects of free radicals within the body. For example, research has shown that people who consume lots of antioxidant-rich plants have lower rates of cancer and heart disease.

Cardiovascular Disease

Cardiovascular disease, or CVD, is an umbrella term that includes disorders of the heart and/or arteries, such as coronary heart disease, stroke, angina (chest pain), myocardial infarction (heart attack), and heart failure.

The biggest risk factors for CVD are hypertension (high blood pressure), obesity, hyperlipidemia (high cholesterol and triglycerides), diabetes, cigarette smoking, and physical inactivity.

Lipids and Hyperlipidemia

Having elevated levels of certain lipids in your blood can spell disaster for your heart. The lipids that most concern doctors are cholesterol and triglycerides.

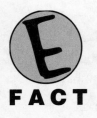

Many experts think that your exposure to stress—and the way you deal with it—can contribute to your susceptibility to cardiovascular disease. Stress can also exacerbate other behaviors that are associated with heart disease (for example, if you're stressed out you might overeat or smoke more than you otherwise would).

Cholesterol is a fat-like substance that your body manufactures (but also occurs in many foods). It's made up of chemicals called *lipoproteins*, which include high-density lipoproteins (HDL) and low-density lipoproteins (LDL). HDL is "good" because it transports cholesterol out of your system. LDL is "bad" because it deposits the cholesterol on the arterial walls. Triglycerides are a different type of fat, also found in your blood and the foods you eat.

High Blood Pressure

Having hypertension increases the amount of work your heart must do, causing it to thicken and become stiff, which increases the chances of heart attack and congestive heart failure. High blood pressure also ups the risk of stroke.

Because hypertension often produces no symptoms, millions of people don't know they have it. In the vast majority of cases, doctors can't identify the cause (this is called *primary hypertension*). But about 5 to 10 percent of cases can be traced to an underlying condition, such as kidney disease, adrenal gland problems, or a congenital heart defect.

This type of high blood pressure, termed *secondary hypertension*, typically appears suddenly and causes bigger problems than primary hypertension. Secondary hypertension can also be caused by certain medications, including birth control pills, cold remedies, decongestants, and over-the-counter (OTC) pain relievers.

Heart Helpers

Conventional medicine has an arsenal of drugs for treating and preventing CVD. Hyperlipidemia is generally treated with statin drugs, such as atorvastatin (Lipitor) and rosuvastatin (Crestor), which decrease production of cholesterol by the liver; other drugs inhibit the absorption of dietary cholesterol and include ezetimibe (Zetia). These medicines can cause abdominal, back, and joint pain, among other things.

Heart disease is treated with drugs like ARBs (angiotensin receptor blockers), ACE (angiotensin converting enzyme) inhibitors, calcium channel blockers, and beta blockers. Side effects can include cough, headaches, dizziness, fatigue, and nausea.

Many edible plants and plant oils have proven heart-protecting benefits, so many doctors advise incorporating them into your diet. For example:

- **Garlic**
  (*Allium sativum*)

  Eating lots of garlicky foods means less heart disease. Taking garlic powder keeps arteries flexible, helps lower blood pressure, and can prevent the damaging oxidation of cholesterol.

- **Pomegranate**
  (*Punica granatum*)

  There's good evidence that drinking pomegranate juice every day can lower your blood pressure and improve other symptoms of CVD, including atherosclerosis (thickening of the arteries).

- **Psyllium** (*Plantago ovata, P. psyllium*)

  Adding a dose of these high-fiber seeds to your diet can significantly reduce your serum cholesterol levels.

- **Soy**
  (*Glycine max*)

  People who replace other dietary protein (such as red meat) with soy can reduce their cholesterol by as much as 10 percent.

- **Tea**
  (*Camellia sinensis*)

  Green tea can lower cholesterol and triglycerides, and research shows that consuming three or more cups a day significantly decreases the risk of cardiovascular and all-cause mortality.

- **Rice bran**
  (*Oryza sativa*)

  Full-fat rice bran and rice bran oil can significantly reduce total cholesterol, LDL, and triglycerides and can increase HDL.

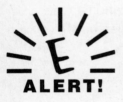
ALERT!

Smoking cigarettes puts you at two to four times the risk of developing coronary heart disease; if you've already got it, you're twice as likely to suffer from sudden cardiac death. Nearly 21 percent of the adults in the United States—or 45.3 million people—are smokers.

Other herbs are used medicinally to treat heart disease. They include:

- **Danshen**
  (*Salvia miltiorrhiza*)

  This annual sage plant is used in China to treat CVD. Research shows it acts as a natural ACE inhibitor and works to lower blood pressure, dilate arteries, and decrease blood clotting.

- **Goji-berry**
  (*Lycium barbarum, L. chinense*)

  These bright-red berries contain a chemical called beta-sitosterol, which has been shown to stop the transport of cholesterol from your gastrointestinal tract to your bloodstream. Goji-berries are also rich in antioxidants.

- **Hawthorn**
  (*Crataegus monogyna, C. oxyacantha*)

  This herb is a proven heart-protector. It can increase exercise tolerance, reduce cholesterol, and relieve shortness of breath in heart patients.

The Epidemic of Diabetes

Diabetes is a chronic, incurable disease involving elevated levels of blood sugar, or *glucose*. Rates of diabetes are skyrocketing. According to the CDC, about 24 million Americans now have diabetes, which is more than three million more than just two years ago; that's nearly 8 percent of the population. What's to blame: a high-calorie, high-fat diet and lack of physical exercise.

Diabetes is a disease involving insulin, which is a hormone produced in the pancreas that regulates glucose. Insulin helps move the sugar from your gastrointestinal tract (it comes from the carbohydrates you eat) to the cells throughout your body.

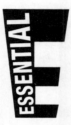

Doctors have identified a milder type of diabetes, known as prediabetes, which involves blood glucose levels that are higher than normal but not as high as a diabetic's. Prediabetes is still serious, however. It significantly increases your risk of developing type 2 diabetes, as well as heart disease and stroke.

There are two main types of diabetes: type 1 (also known as insulin-dependent diabetes), which usually develops in childhood and involves an inability to produce insulin, and type 2 (or adult-onset diabetes), which develops in adulthood. Type 2 is significantly more common—it represents more than 90 percent of all cases of diabetes—and typically begins with *insulin resistance*, a disorder in which the cells stop using insulin properly and continually signal the pancreas to produce more. As the demand rises, the pancreas gradually loses its ability to meet it and full-blown diabetes sets in.

Diabetes is associated with insulin shortfalls, which can be the result of insufficient production, inefficient action, or both.

Without enough insulin, glucose stays in your blood, where it can create short-term problems like fatigue and thirst. Over time, excessive glucose can cause blindness, kidney damage, CVD, and circulatory problems that can lead to lower-limb amputations.

Treatment Options

Conventional medicine treats diabetes with insulin, which is given to some people with type 2 diabetes and everyone with type 1. Diabetics also get oral medications such as metformin (Glucophage, Riomet) and glipizide (Glucotrol), which are hypoglycemics (they lower blood glucose levels); other drugs increase insulin sensitivity and decrease carbohydrate absorption.

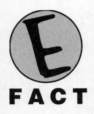

FACT

In recent years, scientists have tied excessive consumption of refined carbohydrates, such as sugar and white bread, with diabetes and insulin resistance. These foods are digested and converted to glucose quickly, which creates a big demand for insulin. Experts advise diabetics and non-diabetics alike to load their plates with unrefined carbohydrates, which don't create blood sugar surges.

People who take insulin (sold under the brand names of Apidra, Humulin, Novolin, and others) can experience mild allergic reactions or low blood sugar, the symptoms of which can include sweating, anxiety, nausea, and rapid heartbeat. Side effects of hypoglycemic drugs can include diarrhea, nausea, stomach pain, and vomiting. Herbal therapies for diabetes, prediabetes, and insulin resistance include these:

- **Cinnamon** (*Cinnamomum verum, C. aromaticum*)   Some studies show that this popular spice can lower blood glucose levels by increasing insulin receptor sensitivity.

- **Fenugreek** (*Trigonella foenum-graecum*)   The seeds of this plant are used as a diabetes remedy in India and other parts of the world. They seem to slow carbohydrate absorption and lower glucose levels.

- **Ginseng** (*Panax ginseng, P. quinquefolius, Eleutherococcus senticosus*)   All of the major varieties of ginseng—Asian, American, and Siberian (eleuthero)—have been shown to lower blood sugar levels.

- **Gymnema**
  (*Gymnema sylvestre*)

  In Hindi, this Indian plant is known as *gur-mar*, or "sugar destroyer." Research shows that diabetics who take a gymnema extract can cut their insulin doses in half and can reduce or even discontinue taking conventional hypoglycemic drugs.

- **Konjac**
  (*Amorphophallus konjac,*
  A. rivieri)

  This tuber, also known as devil's tongue, contains a substance called glucomannan, which is a type of indigestible fiber that can regulate glucose levels in diabetics (it also seems to help reduce cholesterol).

- **Milk thistle**
  (*Silybum marianum*)

  A key chemical constituent in milk thistle, silymarin, has been shown to decrease insulin resistance and stabilize blood sugar and lipid levels in diabetics.

- **Psyllium**
  (*Plantago ovata, P.*
  psyllium)

  Psyllium can significantly lower glucose levels in people with diabetes (both type 1 and type 2).

- **Tulsi** (*Ocimum*
  tenuiflorum, O. sanctum)

  Preliminary research shows that extracts of this Ayurvedic herb can lower blood glucose levels in people with type 2 diabetes.

- **Prickly pear**
  (*Opuntia ficus-indica*)

  Studies show that this cactus, also known as nopal, can significantly reduce blood sugar levels in some type 2 diabetics.

Liver Disease

The liver processes blood as it leaves the stomach and intestines, breaking down nutrients and drugs and filtering out toxins. Chronic liver disease affects one in ten Americans and kills 27,000 of them each year. Any disease of the liver can inhibit its ability to process and eliminate drugs—both pharmaceuticals and medicinal herbs—meaning they can accumulate and reach toxic levels. If you've got any liver issues, talk with your doctor about taking any medicine or supplement, and avoid alcohol (your liver won't be able to process that drug properly, either).

Alcohol-induced Liver Disease

If you regularly drink more alcohol than your liver can handle, the alcohol overload can cause several diseases.

- **Fatty liver disease** affects almost all heavy drinkers and involves the accumulation of excess fat cells. Symptoms can include abdominal discomfort, although many people won't see any signs at all. It will improve if you stop drinking.
- **Alcoholic hepatitis** affects up to 35 percent of heavy drinkers and creates nausea, abdominal pain, fever, and jaundice (a yellowing of your skin and the whites of your eyes). The damage can be reversed if you eliminate the alcohol but can lead to progressive and permanent liver damage if you don't.
- **Alcoholic cirrhosis** affects about 20 percent of heavy drinkers, most often after ten or more years of serious imbibing. In cirrhosis, normal liver tissue is replaced with scar tissue. Symptoms are similar to those of alcoholic hepatitis (see above), but the damage is irreversible.

Infectious Hepatitis

This is caused by a virus—commonly known as hepatitis A, B, or C—and typically produces fever, headache, fever, and jaundice. Symptoms and treatments vary:

- **Hepatitis A** (HVA), which is generally transmitted through contaminated food or water, typically clears up after six months without causing permanent damage.
- **Hepatitis B** (HVB) can be acute (short-term, without any lasting problems) or chronic (ongoing and possibly leading to cirrhosis, cancer, or liver failure). It's transmitted through bodily fluids and from mother to baby during childbirth.
- **Hepatitis C** (HVC) is transmitted via blood and often produces no symptoms (meaning it can go undetected for years). Hepatitis C damages the liver and can lead to potentially fatal liver diseases.

Hepatitis A is generally treated with a vaccine, which can help thwart the infection. Doctors typically let an acute hepatitis B infection run its course without any drug treatments; chronic HVB and HVC infections may be treated with antiviral drugs called *interferons*, which can cause muscle pain and other side effects.

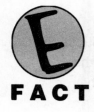

FACT

The most common cause of acute liver failure in the United States is overdosing on acetaminophen (Tylenol). Taking more than the recommended doses or combining the drug with alcohol can create more toxic byproducts than your liver can handle. Excessive doses of other OTC and prescription drugs can also cause liver toxicity.

Herbal Liver Helpers

If you've got liver disease, you should definitely follow your doctor's advice (and take the meds that are prescribed), but you can also use herbs to support your liver and its functioning. For example:

- **Artichoke** (*Cynara cardunculus, C. scolymus*)
Artichoke is a choleretic (it enhances the flow of bile) and rich source of antioxidants. It helps the liver process fats and cholesterol and protects it from oxidative damage.

- **Cordyceps** (*Cordyceps sinensis*)
Extracts of this mushroom can improve liver function in people with infectious hepatitis. It also improves triglyceride and blood sugar levels in diabetics, which could help prevent fatty liver disease.

- **Milk thistle** (*Silybum marianum*)
Milk thistle extracts support liver function and can improve the symptoms of alcoholic liver disease and infectious hepatitis. They also stimulate liver regeneration and the formation of new liver cells.

- **Schisandra** (*Schisandra chinensis*)
Schisandra extracts can protect the liver and have been shown to improve liver function in patients with viral and drug-induced hepatitis.

Cancer

The 100-plus diseases known as cancer share a common cause: the growth and spread of abnormal cells, which are created when the cells' genetic material is mutated though a process called *carcinogenesis*. This upsets the normal balance between the birth and death of cells—termed *apoptosis*—and creates a process of uncontrolled proliferation and tumor formation.

Causes of Cancer

Cancer can be traced to internal factors (genetics, immune conditions, or hormonal problems) and external factors (smoking or exposure to chemicals, radiation, or infectious agents). All of these things can act together or sequentially to create disease.

E-QUESTION

Who is at risk for cancer?
Cancer can strike anyone, but more than three-fourths of all cancers occur in people over fifty-five. When experts talk about risk, they're most often talking about lifetime risk: the likelihood that you'll develop cancer over the course of your lifetime. In the United States, men have a slightly less than 50-percent lifetime risk; for women, it's roughly one in three.

Normally, the cells throughout your body behave in an orderly fashion, growing, dividing, and dying according to schedule (replicating more quickly when you're young and slowing down to replace only worn-out or dying cells as you reach adulthood).

In most cases, if a cell's DNA is damaged, the cell will repair the damage or die. But if the cell survives with a specific mutation, it becomes cancerous. Cancerous cells don't die the way normal cells do; instead, they outlive normal cells and create millions of new cancer cells, which can create tumors and invade other areas of the body, a process called *metastasis*.

The Most Common Cancers

The American Cancer Society estimates that more than 1.4 million Americans were diagnosed with cancer—and 565,000 Americans died—in 2008. Cancer accounts for one in four deaths and claims more than 1,500 lives a day.

Nonmelanoma skin cancer is by far the most common type of cancer in the United States, with more than a million new diagnoses each year (about half of all cancer diagnoses combined). After skin cancer, the most commonly diagnosed cancers, in order of prevalence, are lung, prostate, and colorectal (in men), and breast, lung, and colorectal (in women).

Cancers of the breast and female reproductive system (including the cervix, uterus, and ovaries) kill about 69,000 women every year. Breast cancer accounts for more than one in four cancers diagnosed in American women.

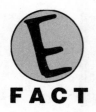

FACT

Lung cancer is the biggest cancer killer in the United States, and the vast majority of cases can be traced to smoking. Tobacco use causes 90 percent of all lung cancer deaths and a significant proportion of deaths from other diseases. It kills 5.4 million people a year—and about half of the people who use it.

Treatment Options

Conventional medical treatment often involves surgical removal of the tumor and other affected tissues, radiation, and chemotherapy (treatment with drugs that kill cancer cells and stop tumor proliferation). In the case of hormone-dependent cancers (prostate cancer in men, breast and reproductive cancers in women), patients may be given hormonal therapies. The side effects of chemotherapy drugs include intense nausea and fatigue; hormonal therapies can increase the risk of other cancers and circulatory and liver problems.

Here are some herbal options, which in many cases can be used in conjunction with conventional treatments:

- **Astragalus** (*Astragalus membranaceus*) — This herb relieves chemotherapy-induced nausea; research shows it can also boost immunity and inhibit tumor growth.

- **Cordyceps** (*Cordyceps sinensis*) — Extracts of the cordyceps mushroom have been shown to reduce tumor size, boost immune response, and improve quality of life in cancer patients.

- **Evening primrose**
  (*Oenothera biennis*)

  This oil can improve the response to the drug tamoxifen in women with breast cancer (it also inhibits the action of a common cancer gene, thus hindering the development of tumors).

- **Ginger**
  (*Zingiber officinale*)

  Ginger extracts can relieve the nausea caused by chemotherapy.

- **Grape**
  (*Vitis vinifera*)

  Red grapes and grape products (wine and juice) contain a potent anticancer chemical called resveratrol. It's also sold as supplements derived from the Japanese knotweed (*Fallopia japonica*) plant. Resveratrol appears to inhibit the growth of cancer cells and to induce apoptosis, and has shown promise in preventing cancer, as well.

- **Reishi**
  (*Ganoderma lucidum*)

  Reishi mushrooms have been used to treat several types of cancer. Studies show that reishi extracts can stimulate immune function in advanced cancer patients and slow the spread of breast, prostate, and other cancer cells.

- **Saw palmetto**
  (*Serenoa repens*)

  Preliminary research has shown that saw palmetto extracts may inhibit the spread of prostate cancer cells and speed their death.

- **Turkey tail**
  (*Trametes versicolor, Coriolus versicolor*)

  Also known as coriolus, this mushroom can prolong cancer survival when taken during chemotherapy or radiation treatment.

- **Tea**
  (*Camellia sinensis*)

  Green tea has been shown to help prevent numerous cancers and also prevent new blood vessel growth in cancers, inhibit tumor cell proliferation, and induce apoptosis in cancer cells.

"Mystery" Diseases

Humans are growing increasingly susceptible to several diseases that, although well known and well researched, remain mysterious. Researchers and doctors can identify the symptoms and even predict the people who are the greatest risk of developing them, yet are at a loss to explain exactly what causes them—or why they're becoming so widespread.

Autoimmune Disorders

Autoimmune disorders are characterized by an abnormal immune response—the body mistakes its own tissues as a threat and attacks them—and can affect any part of the body, including the heart, skin, and endocrine and digestive systems. Some of the most well known are lupus, rheumatoid arthritis (RA), celiac disease, and type 1 diabetes; other diseases that may be linked to autoimmunity include multiple sclerosis and psoriasis.

Autoimmune disorders are the third most common kind of disease in the United States, right behind cancer and heart disease.

Chronic Fatigue Syndrome

Chronic fatigue syndrome, or CFS, was once dismissed as psychosomatic "yuppie flu." CFS is now recognized as a serious health problem that affects more than a million Americans—and it is four times more common in women than men. Symptoms include overwhelming exhaustion, persistent muscle and joint pain, sleep disturbances, headaches, and impaired concentration and memory.

Fibromyalgia

Fibromyalgia is a disorder characterized by widespread pain, abnormal pain processing (sensitivity to things other people wouldn't find painful), fatigue, sleep disturbances, and psychological problems. It affects more than 5 million Americans, mostly women (the ratio of women to men is seven to one).

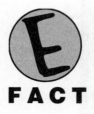

FACT

Fibromyalgia creates "tender points" in the patient's body—on the neck, arms, shoulders, back, hips, and legs—that hurt at the slightest pressure. Like other autoimmune diseases, fibromyalgia is more common in people with rheumatoid arthritis and other immune-related problems or who have a close relative with them.

Conventional and Herbal Treatments

Conventional treatments for autoimmune disorders include pain medications and drugs that treat specific symptoms (i.e., swelling or skin rashes), such as corticosteroids and nonsteroidal anti-inflammatory drugs (NSAIDs). Conventional therapies for CFS include immunomodulating drugs, antivirals, antidepressants, and antianxiety medications. Fibromyalgia is generally treated with NSAIDs, opioids, antidepressants, and muscle relaxants.

Many natural remedies can be used in conjunction with these drugs, although people with autoimmune disorders should avoid taking herbs that stimulate immunity. Safe herbal therapies include:

- **Ashwagandha**
  (*Withania somnifera*)

  This Indian herb is a rich source of antioxidants. Recent research shows it can help offset the oxidative stress that causes many CFS symptoms (and seems to play a role in fibromyalgia, as well).

- **Asian ginseng**
  (*Panax ginseng*)

  This herb can fight fatigue and boost immunity. It is considered an adaptogen, meaning it can help offset the stress that might be behind fibromyalgia and CFS.

- **Astragalus**
  (*Astragalus membranaceus*)

  Also considered adaptogenic, astragalus can calm an overactive immune system—just what you need in an autoimmune disorder. Recent research confirms its modulating effect on immune response in people with systemic lupus.

- **Bilberry**
  (*Vaccinium myrtillus*)

  Bilberry contains antioxidants, which are beneficial in the management of CFS.

- **Cayenne**
  (*Capsicum annuum, C. frutescens*)

  Cayenne is a natural painkiller (and the key ingredient in many OTC arthritis rubs). Research shows it also has immunosuppressive activity and can inhibit inflammation that's caused by an exaggerated immune response. Other studies show it can reduce tenderness and pain in patients with fibromyalgia.

- **Feverfew**
  (*Tanacetum parthenium*)

  Feverfew seems to interact directly with white blood cells to slow the inflammatory process and reduce the severity and frequency of RA episodes.

- **Flax**
  (*Linum usitatissimum*)

  Oral doses of flaxseed have been shown to improve kidney function in people with systemic lupus.

- **Ginger**
  (*Zingiber officinale*)

  Ginger extracts have been shown to decrease joint pain in people with RA.

- **Grape**
  (*Vitis vinifera*)

  Grape seeds and skins contain polyphenols, which are potent anti-inflammatories and antioxidants that can prevent the development of type 1 diabetes and protect cartilage from the damage caused by RA.

CHAPTER 8

Treating Aches and Pains

Herbal remedies are perfect for treating the aches and pains that all people experience at one time or another. Unlike the drugs prescribed by conventional medicine, which typically attack a specific bodily function—inflammation, for example—with a synthetic and single-purpose drug, the medicinal constituents of herbs typically work synergistically, meaning they generally don't have the side effects of pharmaceuticals.

The Anatomy of an Injury

Injuries to the body can take many forms: a contusion or sprain, inflammation from arthritis or tendinitis, a sore back or an aching head brought on by stress. All have one thing in common: irriation or damage to the body's tissues.

Say you're running toward home plate, savoring your imminent triumph (and composing your victory speech in your head) when—wham!—you hit the dirt.

Maybe you pulled a muscle? Or twisted an ankle? Either way, you've done some damage. If the fall was sudden enough, you've probably torn some muscle (or tendon or ligament) fibers, triggering an almost immediate response in your body. Nerves send a pain message to your brain, which in turn tells you to stop what you were doing lest things get any worse. Blood is quickly sent to the injury site, carrying the body's defensive foot soldiers (white blood cells) and stabilizing the area until help arrives. It's the inflammatory response in action.

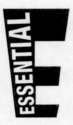

The term *inflammation* applies to more than one condition. Local inflammation is associated with an injury or infection in one part of the body. Systemic inflammation is often tied to multisystem, long-term diseases like lupus. These conditions, known as autoimmune disorders, are the result of the body's immune system mistaking its own cells for foreign invaders.

Now, say you're sitting in your favorite chair, watching the evening news, when you feel an ache in your knee. It's been there for awhile, so long that you hardly notice it anymore. That ache is also the result of inflammation, which in this case is occurring as a result of an old injury. There's no emergency here, no microbial intruders to destroy, but your body is reacting to this trauma in the same way it would to any other: with inflammation.

Although it's the source of countless health problems, inflammation can be a good thing. In inflammation, the body sends blood to the site of some kind of trauma to protect itself from infection or further injury. Signs of inflammation include pain, redness, warmth, and swelling (edema). If the inflammation is happening in a joint or muscle, you'll also experience stiffness and some loss of function.

All of this is good, of course, unless that inflammatory process gets stuck in the "on" position. This can be caused by a few things: Maybe you're perpetuating the damage by continuing to do the things that cause the injury in the first place, or you're developing a chronic condition, like arthritis or bursitis, in which the inflammation is doing nothing but creating more inflammation. Ongoing inflammation can cause any number of problems, but in the case of everyday aches and pains it usually means swelling and discomfort that never go away. It can also mean damage to the tissues in the area, including cartilage and bone.

Herbal Helpers

Herbs generally contain hundreds of ingredients, called *phytochemicals*, many of which have proven pharmacological benefits in treating general aches and pains.

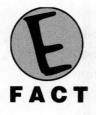

Phytochemicals are usually referred to as *secondary constituents* because they're secondary to the plant's survival. (Primary constituents are involved in the plant's essential metabolic processes.) But it's these nonessentials that are the key to a plant's medicinal value, and scientists generally attribute a plant's bioactivity (its effect on another living organism) to its secondary chemistry.

Chemical Actions

Phytochemicals are most often produced by a plant as a form of self-preservation. Some act like the chemical equivalent of spines on a cactus, defending the plant from the animals, insects, and microbes that otherwise might eat it (or give it a deadly disease). Others protect the plant against environmental stresses like extreme temperatures or drought.

Luckily, phytochemicals can help people, too. Over the millennia, we've discovered plants whose phytochemicals work as antimicrobial agents, astringents, anti-inflammatories, and anesthetics, all of which can help people deal with aches and pains.

Advantages of Herbs Over Drugs

Although they often contain powerful ingredients, herbs are generally considered a gentler form of healing than the pharmaceuticals and procedures of conventional medicine. That's because the side effects of most herbal remedies are rare—and much less troubling than their conventional medicine counterparts.

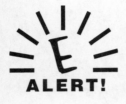

ALERT!

Several new studies have shown that many popular conventional pain medicines can have scary side effects. For example, combining acetaminophen (Tylenol) with large amounts of caffeine could cause liver damage. And migraine sufferers who take the drug topiramate (Topamax) are at a greater risk for kidney stones.

Conventional treatment for most aches and pains typically involves over-the-counter (OTC) nonsteroidal anti-inflammatory drugs (NSAIDs) such as aspirin, naproxen (Aleve), and ibuprofen (Motrin or Advil), and the pain reliever acetaminophen (Tylenol). Some people also use prescription NSAIDs such as celecoxib (Celebrex) to manage chronic pain. But NSAIDs can have serious effects, including stomach bleeding and increased risk of a heart attack. High doses of acetaminophen can lead to liver toxicity.

In cases that involve chronic inflammation in or around a joint (such as bursitis or tendinitis) and don't respond to these drugs, a doctor might prescribe a more powerful anti-inflammatory, such as a corticosteroid (steroidal drug), which can be injected directly into the joint or surrounding area. But while corticosteroids can relieve pain, they can also cause serious side effects, including headaches, elevated blood pressure, muscle weakness, impaired wound healing, ulcers, and psychiatric disturbances. Moreover, steroid drugs can actually damage cartilage and weaken tendons and muscles. This can be especially problematic if the injection was made into a weight-bearing joint, such as the ankle or knee.

Chronic Inflammation

Arthritis, bursitis, and tendinitis are three conditions that share a common culprit: inflammation. When they settle into your joints or other tissues, these conditions can run the gamut from annoying to crippling.

Bursitis

Bursitis is inflammation of the *bursae*, which are small, fluid-filled sacs that keep the bones, tendons, and muscles around your joints cushioned and thus keep the joints moving smoothly. Bursae are also located between bones and other structures (like muscles and skin) that move against the bone. If a bursa becomes inflamed, generally because of overuse or repetitive strain, that movement becomes painful.

Arthritis

Arthritis is the number one cause of disability in the United States. Although arthritis is quite common in seniors—roughly half of everyone over sixty-five has been diagnosed with it—it's not strictly an old-person's disease. Almost two-thirds of the 46 million Americans with diagnosed arthritis are younger than sixty-five.

Arthritis encompasses more than 100 different conditions, but osteoarthritis is the most common, typically striking people who put excessive strain on their joints, have had a joint injury (or joint malformation), are overweight, or have a family history of the disease.

Technically speaking, osteoarthritis isn't caused by inflammation; it comes from physical wear and tear. However, because osteoarthritis includes joint pain, swelling, and loss of function—all symptoms of inflammation—it's is generally lumped in with the rest.

Tendinitis

Tendinitis (or tendonitis) is an inflammation in the tendon, which is the fibrous, cord-like material that joins muscle to bone. It's caused by repetitive strain or injury—think tennis elbow and swimmer's shoulder—but it's not reserved for athletes: Painting or shoveling also can trigger it, as can using incorrect posture or neglecting to stretch before activity.

Tendinitis produces pain just outside the affected joint. Adults over forty are more susceptible, because tendons become less flexible and more injury-prone as you age.

Treatment Options

The "itis" conditions are typically treated with OTC or prescription medicines such as NSAIDs. But there are several herbs that can treat pain, stiffness, and inflammation without the side effects.

- **Ashwagandha** (*Withania somnifera*)

  Research shows that this Indian herb can deliver significant and sustained pain relief, alleviate stiffness, and restore function to arthritic joints.

- **Cat's claw** (*Uncaria guianensis, U. tomentosa*)

  Studies have confirmed that this South American plant—traditionally used as an anti-inflammatory—is useful against osteoarthritis.

- **Pineapple** (*Ananas comosus*)

  Pineapples contain bromelain, an enzyme that's used to treat inflammation. Research shows that bromelain, used alone or in combination therapies, can reduce swelling and manage the pain and inflammation of arthritis.

- **Rose hip** (*Rosa canina, R. spp.*)

  Recent research has shown that powdered rose hip, which contains high levels of vitamin C, can decrease pain and stiffness in arthritis.

- **Turmeric** (*Curcuma longa*)

  Turmeric can block inflammation and prevent arthritis-related bone loss. In one study, turmeric and frankincense (*Boswellia serrata*) significantly reduced pain in patients with arthritic knees.

Back Pain

Whether it's an ache in the lower back or a twinge in the neck, back pain is the most widespread orthopedic condition in the United States, affecting about 80 percent of people.

Back pain is really not a condition—it's a symptom of an underlying problem in the muscles, nerves, and/or bones of the spine. In many cases, it's a sign of a mechanical problem, such as muscle tension: Maybe you've put undue strain on your back by lifting a heavy object improperly, suddenly twisting your back or neck, or maintaining poor posture for a long time while sitting or standing.

Another mechanical problem is a condition known as intervertebral disk degeneration, which is breakdown of the disks located between the bones, or vertebrae, of your spine. Back pain can also be the result of an injury or a condition like scoliosis (a curvature of the spine) or arthritis.

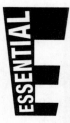

Sciatica is a type of back pain that involves the sciatic nerve, which runs from the lower back into the legs. Symptoms can include shooting pain, numbness, or tingling in the backside and one leg. Sciatica can occur during pregnancy, and it is also more common in people who are overweight and inactive. Wearing high heels or sleeping on a mattress that is too soft can also contribute to sciatica.

Treatment Options

Conventional medicine treats back pain in a few ways, depending on its cause and severity. For most minor cases, you'll be advised to take NSAIDs and try physical therapy, massage, or controlled exercise. If you're experiencing serious or chronic back pain (lasting longer than six weeks), be sure to talk with your health care provider.

Several herbs have been used traditionally to treat back pain—and are showing their abilities in modern laboratories as well. For example:

- **Cramp bark** (*Viburnum opulus*)
  Also known as guelder rose (among other names), this is a key Western herbal remedy for muscle cramps; it is effective against spasmodic back pain (it has analgesic, antispasmodic, and anti-inflammatory properties).

- **Devil's claw** (*Harpagophytum procumbens*)
  This is a classic South African remedy for pain and inflammation. Research shows that an oral extract can significantly reduce back pain.

- **Ginger** (*Zingiber officinale*)
  Ginger, which is an analgesic and anti-inflammatory, is used both topically and internally to treat muscle and joint pain. Modern research shows it works like the NSAIDs to reduce inflammation.

- **Lavender**
  (*Lavandula
  angustifolia*)

  The aromatic essential oil is a traditional remedy used to relax both muscles and mind. It's been proven effective at reducing stress as well as pain and inflammation.

- **Willow**
  (*Salix alba*)

  The bark from this tree contains salicin, a precursor of aspirin. Research has shown it to be an effective analgesic and a powerful weapon against back pain. In one study, willow extracts relieved pain better than the prescription drug rofecoxib (Vioxx).

Muscle Aches, Sprains, and Strains

Anytime you ask a muscle to do something that it's not used to doing (such as running ten extra miles or lifting extra-heavy weights), the muscle can respond with pain. Muscle pain also can be caused by an acute injury, such as a fall, or chronic (also known as overuse) injuries. It can range from mild (a dull ache or twinge) to intense (significant pain or stiffness).

Sprains and strains are some of the most common sports injuries. A *sprain* is an injury to the ligaments, which are the fibrous bands that attach muscle to bone. A *strain* is an injury to a muscle or tendon, which is the structure that attaches a muscle to another muscle. Both sprains and strains occur when the tissue is stretched (or torn) because it's been pulled past its normal range of motion.

ESSENTIAL

Conventional treatment for sprains and strains uses what the experts call PRICE: protect, rest, ice, compression, and elevation. That means you immediately stop using the affected joint (protect it and give it a rest), apply ice or a cold pack and gentle compression (via an elastic wrap), and elevate the joint, all of which will help reduce the swelling.

If you sprain something, you'll know it. In some cases, you'll hear a popping sound as the ligaments are overextended. In all cases, you'll experience almost immediate swelling and pain. You should see a doctor if these symptoms are severe (if you can't put any weight at all on the ankle, for example).

If you've sustained a strain (what many people call a "pulled muscle"), you'll feel immediate pain and increasing stiffness (and possible swelling) over the next few hours. The most common cause of strains are sudden, powerful contractions of a muscle group—like when you slip and fall on the ice, lunge to return a tennis shot, or jump to sink a basket.

Herbal Helpers

To fight the pain of most muscle injuries, you can skip the NSAIDs in favor of these herbal remedies:

- **Arnica** (*Arnica montana*) — Arnica is a classic remedy for all kinds of aches, including the sports-induced kind. Studies have confirmed its use as a remedy for soft-tissue (i.e., muscle) injuries.

- **Cayenne** (*Capsicum annuum, C. frutescens*) — These peppers contain a chemical called capsaicin, which can be applied topically to produce a warming sensation and reduce pain (it's the key ingredient in many OTC muscle rubs).

- **Comfrey** (*Symphytum officinale*) — This herb is used topically to treat all kinds of sports injuries, including injuries to muscles, tendons, and ligaments.

- **Eucalyptus** (*Eucalyptus globulus*) — The oil from this Australian plant is used topically as an analgesic and anesthetic.

- **Peppermint** (*Mentha x piperita*) — Peppermint contains menthol, a natural anesthetic and painkiller. Menthol also produces a soothing, cooling sensation.

- **Pineapple** (*Ananas comosus*) — Pineapple's active constituent, bromelain, can be taken internally to treat a variety of sports injuries and trauma. Studies have shown that it can reduce inflammation, swelling, and bruising.

- **Saint John's wort** (*Hypericum perforatum*) — This herb produces an oil that's used topically to treat muscle and joint injuries (it's got analgesic, antiedemic, and anesthetic constituents). It also works as an anti-inflammatory and antispasmodic.

- **Yarrow** (*Achillea millefolium*) — Yarrow relieves pain and swelling and is a classic remedy for swelling, bruising, and muscle soreness.

Headaches

Seven in ten Americans have at least one headache a year, and 45 million people live with chronic headaches. Headaches can go from merely annoying to debilitating, and the term *headache* encompasses at least twelve major types, including tension headaches, caffeine-withdrawal headaches, hunger headaches, menstrual headaches, hangover headaches, and ice cream headaches (a.k.a. "brain freeze").

Tension-type Headaches

Also known as ordinary or idiopathic headaches, these involve infrequent, episodic pain that can last from a few minutes to a few days. The pain is usually bilateral (meaning it's on both sides of your head) and accompanies a sensation of pressure or tightening. This is the most common type of headache, experienced by roughly 78 percent of the population. Most often, tension headaches are treated with NSAIDs or acetaminophen.

Sinus Headaches

As the name implies, these are created from pressure in the sinus cavities, which may be caused by congestion from a cold or allergies or inflammation from an infection (if you've got an infection, you'll probably have a fever as well). Sinus headaches are generally treated with NSAIDs, antihistamines, and decongestants—plus antibiotics in the case of sinus infection.

Cluster Headaches

These are rare and are extremely intense; they tend to "cluster" over a period of weeks or months, only to go away and reappear later. Cluster headaches typically come on a few times a day and last about forty-five minutes. They occur more often in young men and in people who frequently smoke and drink alcohol. Conventional medical treatment for cluster headaches typically includes drugs like sumatriptan (Imitrex), zolmitriptan (Zomig), or rizatriptan (Maxalt), which are used to prevent a headache or stop one that's already started. Side effects include tightness in the chest and dizziness.

Migraine Headaches

Migraines are intense and pounding and often accompanied by visual disturbances (called *auras*), sensitivity to light and noise, nausea, and vomiting. Every year, about 30 million people in the United States experience a migraine.

As with cluster headaches, conventional migraine treatments involve acute and preventive measures. In patients with mild to moderate attacks, NSAIDs are generally recommended. More severe cases are given prescription NSAIDs like naproxen (Naprosyn). Preventive and treatment meds include sumatriptan (Imitrex), zolmitriptan (Zomig), or rizatriptan (Maxalt).

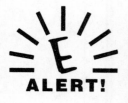

ALERT!

Migraine pain causes many sufferers to try almost anything for relief. A recent national survey found that 20 percent of people who suffer from regular migraine headaches routinely take dangerous, potentially addictive medications that contain barbiturates or opioids (and have not been approved by the FDA) in their quest for a cure.

Herbal Headache Relief

Many traditional herbal formulas have shown the ability to handle even the toughest of headaches:

- **Butterbur** (*Petasites hybridus*) — Extracts from this shrub have analgesic, anti-inflammatory, and antiseizure actions. In several recent studies, they produced a marked decrease in severity and frequency of migraines.

- **Cayenne** (*Capsicum annuum, C. frutescens*) — Applied topically, cayenne preparations have been shown to relieve and even prevent the devastating pain of cluster headaches.

- **Feverfew** (*Tanacetum parthenium*) — This is perhaps the best-known herbal headache remedy. It has been shown in several studies to reduce the frequency of migraine attacks—and limit their symptoms when they do occur.

- **Lavender** (*Lavandula angustifolia*) — The essential oil of this flowering plant has been used effectively to treat several types of headache pain. The same is true of peppermint oil (*Mentha x piperita*).

- **Willow** (*Salix alba*) — The salicin from the bark of this tree is a potent analgesic. Its headache-fighting properties are well proven in both laboratory and clinical studies.

CHAPTER 9

Taming Allergies and Asthma

Allergies and asthma are everywhere: Roughly 45 million Americans have allergies, which are exaggerated immune system reactions to benign things like pollen and cat fur. And close to 20 million Americans have asthma, a chronic disease involving the respiratory system (and often the immune system, as well). Both conditions are growing increasingly common, leading experts to think that our environment may be contributing to the problem—and conventional medical treatments aren't doing much to stop it.

What's Behind the Symptoms?

Allergies are the result of an exaggerated immune response to an agent, or *allergen*, that's not really dangerous but is treated as such by the body's defenses. Allergies are closely related to atopic dermatitis and asthma, two other conditions in which the immune system overreacts to a harmless trigger.

The term *allergies* applies to several distinct diseases, all with their own symptoms and treatments. However, they have a common underlying cause: a hypersensitivity to otherwise benign things. Some of the most common allergic conditions are:

- Allergic rhinitis, also known as hay fever or nasal allergies
- Allergic asthma, a type of asthma triggered by an allergic reaction
- Insect bite/sting allergies
- Skin allergies
- Food allergies
- Drug allergies
- Eye allergies, also known as allergic conjunctivitis

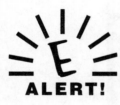

Some herbs used to treat allergies and asthma can cause allergic reactions themselves in sensitive individuals. Anyone who's allergic to plants in the *Asteraceae/Compositae* family, which include ragweed and daisies, should avoid remedies made with other family members, such as arnica (*Arnica montana*), butterbur (*Petasites hybridus*), calendula (*Calendula officinalis*), chamomile (*Matricaria recutita*), echinacea (*Echinacea purpurea*), and yarrow (*Achillea millefolium*).

Some of these conditions overlap: Food allergies can trigger an allergic reaction in the skin as well as in the digestive tract, for example, and inhaled irritants that can trigger an episode of allergic rhinitis might also bring on allergic asthma.

The Allergic Response

Allergic symptoms typically include inflammation. In the case of allergic rhinitis, that can mean itchiness (in the eyes and nose and possibly the skin in other parts of your body), sneezing, and a runny nose. If the airways are irritated, symptoms can also include coughing, wheezing, and shortness of breath. In skin reactions, you might develop red patches, hives, or a rash.

An allergic response is a misguided reaction of your immune system to something that doesn't present a threat (and doesn't bother other people, unless they happen to be allergic to the same thing).

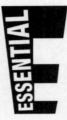

Many people treat the sniffles caused by nasal allergies with nonprescription decongestant nasal sprays. But overuse of these sprays can make things worse, creating a chronic condition known as nonallergic rhinitis. That happens when the tissues in your nasal passages become conditioned to the chemicals in the spray, causing you to use more and more to get the same results.

Allergies are caused by a complex process that can be traced back to an antibody called *immunoglobulin E*, or IgE, which the body releases in response to a trigger (a substance to which it's been exposed before and is now sensitized). In the bloodstream, IgE antibodies bind to mast cells, which are located in the tissues that line the nose, bronchial tubes, gastrointestinal tract, and skin. This triggers the release of chemicals called *mediators* (including histamine and leukotrienes) and sets off a chain reaction that produces the classic "allergic" reaction. IgEs are the key to allergies. If your immune system produces IgEs whenever it encounters cats (or more precisely, proteins from the cat's skin), you'll be allergic to cats.

Most experts think that both environment and genetics play a role in who'll develop allergic conditions. Allergies run in families, and research shows that people with allergies are more likely to develop asthma. Allergies are also closely tied to dermatitis, and people with allergic asthma and certain allergies—or who have family members with allergic conditions—are more likely to develop dermatitis.

Conventional Versus Herbal Treatments

Conventional medicine tackles allergic conditions in two ways: by individually treating symptoms of an acute allergy (or asthma) attack and attempting to prevent or minimize future attacks. These treatments focus almost entirely on symptom management—shutting down the body's reactions to triggers by suppressing the individual functions. For example, nasal allergy sufferers are given antihistamines to avert the sniffling-and-sneezing symptoms of an allergic reaction. Asthmatics are given steroid medications that reduce inflammation in the airways.

Although they have their drawbacks, the conventional drugs that are used to treat these conditions are valuable in many cases—and essential in serious ones. However, herbs can be used quite effectively, alone or as a support for conventional medications. For example, herbal remedies can be used safely to relieve congestion in the upper and lower respiratory tracts, relax spasms, and soothe inflamed tissues in the airways. Herbal remedies also work to support the body's immunity and other functions.

Allergic Rhinitis

Also known as hay fever, allergic rhinitis is the most common type of allergic reaction. If it is caused by outdoor irritants, such as pollen from trees or grasses, it is labeled a seasonal allergy. When it's triggered by things that are present year-round, allergic rhinitis is designated as perennial. This type of allergy is generally caused by indoor irritants, such as pet dander (dandruff-like material that collects in the animal's fur), dust mites (tiny insects that live in pillows and other soft goods in your house), mold, and cockroach droppings.

Typical Symptoms

Rhinitis—which means "inflammation of the nose"—occurs when the nasal membranes become irritated and start producing excessive mucus. Mucus is the fluid produced naturally to trap dust and other particles in the nose and keep them out of the lungs; it's usually thin and barely noticeable as it drains down the back of your throat. In a case of rhinitis, mucus becomes thick and plentiful—clogging things up and draining quite noticeably out the front of your nose. Plain old rhinitis is the stuffiness you get with a cold (this is called *infectious rhinitis*). Allergic rhinitis is what happens when you encounter an allergen.

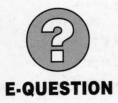

E-QUESTION

How can I tell if I have a cold or allergies?
Sometimes, it can be tough to tell. But generally speaking, you'll know it's an allergic reaction by your nose (allergies produce clear mucus; colds and flu create yellowish discharge), your temperature (allergies won't produce a fever), and the duration of your symptoms (colds and flu clear up within about a week, while allergies disappear as soon as the trigger is gone—and hang around as long as the allergen does).

Pharmaceutical Treatments

The most popular conventional treatments for allergic rhinitis are over-the-counter (OTC) decongestants and antihistamines. Decongestants treat congestion by constricting the blood vessels in the nasal cavities, thereby reducing the amount of mucus that gets into your nose. Antihistamines block the actions of histamine, thereby relieving your runny nose, itchy eyes, and sneezing.

For mild to moderate symptoms, your doctor might suggest OTC decongestants like pseudoephedrine (Sudafed) or short-acting antihistamines, like OTC loratadine (Claritin) and diphenhydramine (Benadryl). Your doctor might also prescribe longer-acting antihistamines, like fexofenadine (Allegra) and Cetirizine (Zyrtec), as well as a nasal spray, azelastine (Astelin).

Some doctors recommend an OTC spray, cromolyn sodium (Nasal-Crom), which is a mast cell stabilizer that prevents the release of histamine.

Another type of nasal allergy treatment, immunotherapy (or allergy shots), is used to desensitize you to allergens. In immunotherapy, you'll be given a series of injections, each containing a slightly higher dose of the allergen that's causing your problems.

For cases that don't respond to decongestants and antihistamines, some doctors prescribe a leukotriene inhibitor, such as montelukast (Singulair), which blocks the substances that trigger allergic (and asthmatic) responses.

Other pharmaceuticals used to treat serious allergies are corticosteroids, including skin creams and nasal sprays such as fluticasone (Flonase) and mometasone (Nasonex).

Herbal Remedies

If you'd rather skip the drugs (or limit your dependence on them), you can alleviate some of the symptoms of allergic rhinitis with these herbs:

- **Butterbur** (*Petasites hybridus*) — Butterbur is traditionally used to treat allergies, coughs, and congestion (it inhibits both histamine and leukotriene release). Recent research has shown that a butterbur extract is as effective as the drugs cetirizine (Zyrtec) or fexofenadine (Allegra) in treating seasonal nasal allergies.

- **Echinacea** (*Echinacea purpurea*) — Echinacea is the go-to remedy for the common cold, and research shows it can lessen the severity of allergic rhinitis, too.

- **Nettle** (*Urtica dioica*) — Nettle is a classic hay fever remedy throughout Europe. It acts like a mast cell stabilizer to stop runny nose and other allergic rhinitis symptoms.

- **Tinospora** (*Tinospora cordifolia*) — Also known as guduchi, this is a classic Indian remedy for allergic rhinitis. It's been shown in recent research to provide significant relief from sneezing, itchy eyes, and other symptoms. It also acts as an immunostimulant, making it an effective form of immunotherapy.

Skin Allergies

Some allergies cause symptoms in your skin. The most common are atopic dermatitis (a chronic condition that produces red, itchy patches) and urticaria (which produces itchy, raised bumps). These reactions can be caused by many things, including something you've inhaled or eaten. A third type of skin allergy is contact dermatitis, which is triggered by direct contact with an allergenic substance.

Atopic Dermatitis

Dermatitis, also known as eczema, is a broad term encompassing many types of skin inflammation. The most common is atopic dermatitis, a chronic, itchy condition in which the skin is overly sensitive to certain triggers. Although it's technically not an allergy, atopic dermatitis primarily affects allergy-prone people and often accompanies other allergic conditions. More than 15 million Americans have it.

Atopic dermatitis most often affects children and babies (see Chapter 6). Although there's no known cause, there are several "triggers" that can cause flare-ups. These include:

- Allergens, such as pollen or mold
- Irritants, such as certain fabrics, soaps, chlorine, or cigarette smoke
- Certain foods, especially eggs, peanuts, and milk
- Other factors, like stress, high temperatures, and low humidity

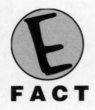

FACT

According to the National Institutes of Health, roughly 2.5 percent of Americans under the age of sixty-five have atopic dermatitis. But this relatively rare condition costs between roughly $600 and $1,250 per patient, per year—representing more than a quarter of the average patient's health care costs. All that adds up to more than $1 billion annually.

Urticaria

Urticaria is a fancy name for hives, a condition that affects about 20 percent of the population at one time or another. Most often, urticaria appears suddenly and disappears a few hours later. In some people, however, the hives stick around much longer, or go away only to reappear a short time later. The most common triggers for urticaria are certain medications, foods, and insect bites.

Contact Dermatitis

If your skin encounters an allergen, you might develop contact dermatitis, in which the affected skin turns red and itchy (as it would after touching poison ivy). Experts have identified more than 3,000 allergens that can cause allergic contact dermatitis. They include: OTC antibiotic creams and ointments, fragrances in many skin and hair care products (even products labeled "unscented" can contain fragrance), and metals such as the nickel in jewelry and the mercury in dental fillings.

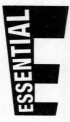

Occasionally, a substance won't cause an allergic response unless it's triggered by something else, such as sunlight (these reactions are called *photoallergies*). This can be the case with skin preparations and some medications. Other people will react to an allergen only after they begin to perspire.

Treatments

Conventional medicine generally treats allergic skin reactions with pharmaceuticals designed to stop the symptoms, if not the reaction itself. These include:

- Topical antihistamines and corticosteroids, which control itching and swelling
- Topical immunomodulating drugs to reduce the immune system's response
- Oral or topical antibiotics to treat infection in inflamed skin
- Oral or injectable corticosteroids
- Oral immunomodulators

Each of these drugs has potential side effects. The last two, which are generally reserved for cases that haven't responded to the other drugs, can cause serious problems, including hypertension and kidney problems. Herbal medicine has some effective alternatives:

- **Astragalus** (*Astragalus membranaceus*)

  Astragalus is used in traditional Eastern medicine to treat all sorts of allergic diseases. In the lab, it's been shown to suppress atopic dermatitis.

- **Hops** (*Humulus lupulus*)

  Native Americans used this herb as a multipurpose skin remedy. New research shows that drinking a hop extract can inhibit all sorts of allergic reactions, including atopic dermatitis.

- **Oats**
  (*Avena sativa*)

  Used in baths and skin care treatments, oatmeal relieves itching and inflammation and creates a barrier to help skin heal.

- **Saint John's wort**
  (*Hypericum perforatum*)

  Saint John's wort is a traditional remedy for many skin problems. Used topically, it inhibits inflammation-building enzymes to relieve atopic dermatitis.

- **Tea**
  (*Camellia sinensis*)

  Tea contains phytochemicals that have been proven effective at suppressing all types of allergic response, including inflammatory skin diseases.

Food Allergies

Roughly 12 million Americans have diagnosed food allergies, a condition in which the immune system reacts to the ingestion of a trigger food by creating inflammation in various parts of the body. Food allergies can trigger symptoms in the digestive system as well as the skin and respiratory tract. True food allergies affect about 7 percent of U.S. children and 2 percent of adults. Typical symptoms of food allergy are:

- Swelling and an itchy sensation in mouth and throat
- Abdominal pain (cramping, bloating)
- Diarrhea
- Nausea and vomiting
- Skin rash
- Coughing or shortness of breath

Most often, a food allergy makes you uncomfortable. However, in rare cases, an allergenic food will trigger a potentially life-threatening condition called *anaphylaxis*, which is an immediate reaction that can cause loss of consciousness and death. Every year, about 30,000 people go into anaphylactic shock caused by a food allergy, and 150 people die from it.

Identify—and Avoid

Because there's no cure for food allergies (and no magical antidote that you can take once you've eaten something allergenic), the only way to avoid an allergic reaction is to avoid the foods that might cause it. While food allergies are more common in children (and typically disappear as the child grows up), allergies to peanuts, nuts, and seafood seldom go away.

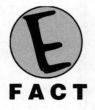

Lots of people who think they have food allergies actually have food intolerances. A true food allergy typically involves a reaction in the skin as well as the digestive system. If you've eaten a food to which you're allergic, symptoms may appear right away—within a few minutes—or may take up to two hours to appear. Food intolerances produce digestive symptoms only.

There are more than 200 foods and food ingredients that can provoke an allergic reaction, but the vast majority are caused by nuts (walnuts, almonds, and pecans), legumes (peanuts and soybeans), milk, eggs, fish, shellfish, and wheat.

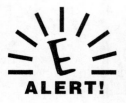

It's fairly easy to avoid allergenic foods—when you can see them. But restaurant meals and manufactured foods often contain potential triggers like milk, soy, and egg whites (which won't be listed on the label if they're part of a flavoring or coloring agent). If you're severely allergic, even a tiny amount can cause a reaction.

Herbal Helpers

If you've had an allergic reaction to a food, you can use a few herbal remedies to help relieve the symptoms:

- **Chamomile**
  (*Matricaria recutita*)

  This herb works as an anti-inflammatory and is useful as a tea and a topical remedy. Research shows it can relieve itching triggered by a food allergy just as well as pharmaceutical preparations.

- **Ginger**
  (*Zingiber officinale*)

  Ginger is a proven stomach-settler that appears to "deactivate" the inflammatory response in laboratory tests.

- **Peppermint**
  (*Mentha x piperita*)

  Peppermint soothes digestive tissues and appears to have an antihistamine-like effect. Research shows it can be effective against stomach upset (including bloating and mild gastrointestinal spasms), cramping, nausea, and vomiting.

- **Rooibos**
  (*Aspalathus linearis*)

  Research shows that rooibos works as a bronchodilator and antispasmodic.

- **Witch hazel**
  (*Hamamelis virginiana*)

  This is a classic skin remedy that relieves allergic itching and inflammation.

Asthma

Asthma is a chronic disease that's generally divided into two types: allergic (or extrinsic) or nonallergic (intrinsic). Of the two, allergic asthma is the most common, affecting about 60 percent of all asthmatics.

Various Triggers

Nonallergic asthma, as the name implies, is not associated with an allergic response. It shares the same symptoms—coughing, wheezing, and difficulty breathing, all caused by inflammation and airway obstruction—but is triggered by things like stress, exercise, and cold or dry air. Thus, it doesn't involve the immune system.

Allergic asthma, on the other hand, is caused by the same kind of overblown immune response that's behind allergies. It's triggered by inhaled allergens, such as dust mites, pet dander, mold, and pollen.

Conventional Treatments for Asthma

There's no cure for asthma (either the allergic or nonallergic kind), and treatments focus on managing symptoms and making attacks less frequent and intense. Western medicine prescribes two types of asthma drugs: long-acting control (or preventive) and short-acting (or emergency).

Long-term control medicines make the airways less sensitive and less reactive, and reduce coughing and wheezing. These drugs include:

- Inhaled anti-inflammatories, including nonsteroidals (or mast cell stabilizers) and corticosteroids
- Beta-agonist bronchodilators (inhaled or taken orally), relax the smooth muscle surrounding the bronchial tubes
- Leukotriene modifiers, which act on chemicals that trigger inflammation and mucus production to reduce swelling and keep the airways open
- Injectable anti-IgE therapy, which prevents the IgE antibodies from binding to mast cells and producing an allergic reaction; this is used in people with moderate to severe allergic asthma

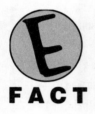

FACT

Herbs can also prevent allergies and asthma. A recent study found that children who eat lots of tomatoes, eggplants, green beans, and zucchini have much lower rates of asthma. Other studies show that babies born to women who regularly eat vegetables (along with fish and legumes) have fewer allergic conditions.

Short-acting, or emergency, medications reduce symptoms during an asthma attack. They include:

- Inhaled beta-agonist bronchodilators, which relax the muscles in and around the airways
- Oral corticosteroids, which are generally reserved for severe cases that don't respond to the other short-term drugs

The list of potential side effects for these drugs is a long one. For example, corticosteroid inhalers can cause hoarseness and thrush (a fungal infection of the mouth). Beta-agonist bronchodilators can cause nervousness, increased heart rate, and insomnia.

Herbal Asthma Alternatives

Herbs that have been used successfully to treat asthma include:

- **Boswellia**
  (*Boswellia serrata*)

  This Ayurvedic herb, also known as Indian frankincense, is taken internally to combat inflammation and has shown antiasthma potential. In one study, people who took oral extracts saw a significant improvement in their symptoms.

- **Coffee**
  (*Coffea arabica*)

  The caffeine in coffee, which is also found in many other herbs—including guarana (*Paullinia cupana*), mate (*Ilex paraguariensis*), and tea (*Camellia sinensis*)—can improve airway function for up to four hours in people with asthma. Chemically speaking, caffeine is related to the asthma drug theophylline; it's a bronchodilator that also reduces fatigue in the respiratory muscles.

- **Eucalyptus**
  (*Eucalyptus globulus*)

  Eucalyptus has analgesic, anti-inflammatory, and mucolytic properties (meaning it destroys mucus). In one study, people with severe asthma who were given oral doses of eucalyptus extract were able to cut back on their use of oral steroids.

- **Ginkgo**
  (*Ginkgo biloba*)

  Ginkgo contains phytochemicals that block the exaggerated immune response that characterizes asthma. Research shows it's effective at dilating the bronchial tubes to keep breathing normal; it's also useful for long-term management of asthma and its associated inflammation.

- **Grapefruit**
  (*Citrus paradisi*)

  Grapefruit and other citrus fruits are high in antioxidants (including vitamin C), and research shows that consuming lots of them can improve lung function and reduce wheezing in asthmatic people.

- **Maritime pine**
  (*Pinus pinaster*)

  Pine bark is a powerful antioxidant and a traditional remedy for coughs and bronchitis. Research has shown that it reduces the severity of symptoms of mild to moderate asthma.

CHAPTER 10

Managing Psychological and Emotional Issues

Psychological (or neuropsychiatric) conditions—a broad term that encompasses cognitive (thinking), emotional, mood, social, and behavioral disorders—can range from mild to debilitating. These problems cause distress and reduce your ability to function professionally, psychologically, socially, and/or interpersonally. Conventional medicine typically treats psychological and emotional disorders with drugs, which can deliver a long list of side effects. But in many cases, herbs can offer a gentler, no less effective type of relief.

A Complex Problem

Modern medicine has come a long way in its understanding of the brain and the disorders that affect it. While earlier generations thought that neuro-psychiatric disorders were best treated radically—with surgery, perhaps, or confinement in an asylum—we now know that mental illnesses, while they are centered in the brain, are quite often the result of biological, psychological, and social factors.

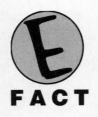

FACT

The National Institutes of Health estimates that more than 62 percent of Americans over the age of eighteen—one in four adults—has a diagnosable mental disorder. Serious disorders like depression, bipolar disorder, and drug dependence cost at least $193 billion annually in lost earnings alone and affect about 6 percent of U.S. adults—or one in every seventeen people.

Types of Disorders

Experts divide mental illnesses into a few categories, including:

- **Mood Disorders** include major depression and bipolar disorder and involve persistent feelings of sadness. In bipolar disorder (sometimes termed manic-depressive disorder), the feelings of sadness alternate with a sense of euphoria or mania.
- **Anxiety Disorders** are characterized by excessive nervousness or anticipation of disaster or danger, along with a general feeling of uncertainty. Anxiety disorders include phobias (such as a fear of heights or closed spaces), panic disorder, obsessive-compulsive disorder (OCD), and post-traumatic stress disorder (PTSD).
- **Developmental Disorders** are problems that generally appear in childhood or infancy, and include autism and attention deficit hyperactivity disorder (ADHD).
- **Substance Abuse Disorders** are centered on the abuse of alcohol and illicit drugs as well as prescription and over-the-counter (OTC) medications and substances like nicotine.

- **Cognitive Disorders** affect your reasoning and thinking. They include dementia, memory disorders, and Alzheimer's disease.
- **Stress**, which involves heightened responses to the challenges of daily life that can produce psychological as well as physical symptoms.

The Mind/Body Connection

As a component of holistic medicine, herbalism is rooted in the belief that the mind and body are inextricably connected, both in sickness and in health. Thus, problems in the physical body often manifest themselves psychologically, and vice versa.

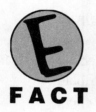

FACT

While psychological and emotional problems affect both genders, women are twice as likely to suffer from depression, post-traumatic stress disorder (PTSD), and panic disorder, in part because their bodies synthesize significantly less of the brain chemical serotonin, required for the healthy maintenance of moods. Women also seem to be more prone to addictions to alcohol, tobacco, and illicit drugs.

Indeed, conventional medical research supports the theory that mind and body work hand in hand, and many studies have found a link between mental and physical diseases. For example:

- *Asthma is connected to depression and anxiety.* A recent study found that teenagers with asthma are twice as likely to have depression or anxiety disorders than the teens without asthma. Other research has shown that asthmatic kids are more likely to have ADHD and other behavioral problems.
- *Depression and anxiety are tied to heart disease.* Research has shown that having either problem doubles your risk of developing coronary artery disease.
- *Migraines are linked to mental disorders.* People who suffer from migraine headaches are more than twice as likely to have mental

disorders such as major depression, bipolar disorder, panic disorder, and social phobia.

- *Diabetes is linked to Alzheimer's disease.* Having diabetes ups the risk of developing Alzheimer's (the same holds true for high blood pressure and high cholesterol). Other research has found a connection between certain viral and bacterial infections and Alzheimer's.
- *Obesity can lead to mental illness.* A recent study found that obese adults were up to twice as likely to suffer from depression, anxiety, dementia, and other mental problems. Another study found that obesity can up your risk of dementia by as much as 80 percent.

Conventional Versus Herbal Treatment

Conventional medicine typically deals with mental disorders with a two-pronged approach: cognitive-behavioral therapy and drug treatment.

Cognitive-behavior therapy, also known as "talk therapy," is based on changing the behaviors, beliefs, and patterns of thinking that can contribute to problems like depression and phobias. Cognitive therapy can also help people manage feelings of shyness, anxiety, or anger.

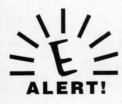

Some conventional drugs can trigger psychological problems. For example, OTC decongestants often cause nervousness, the prescription acne drug isotretinoin (Accutane) can create depression and psychosis, and clarithromycin (Biaxin), an antibiotic, can cause hallucinations, nightmares, and manic behavior. In fact, the FDA is investigating a possible association between montelukast sodium (Singulair), a popular asthma and allergy drug, and suicidal behavior.

Drug Treatments

In many cases, conventional medicine treats mental disorders pharmaceutically. Most of the drugs used to treat mental problems fall into these categories:

- Antipsychotic medications
- Antimanic (or mood-stabilizing) medications
- Antidepressants
- Antianxiety medications
- Stimulants

Herbs: The Natural Alternative

While pharmaceutical interventions are certainly useful—and in some cases, essential—in treating psychological and emotional problems, many can be replaced or augmented with herbal remedies.

Many psychological and emotional problems respond well to herbal treatments—and some conventional doctors and mental health professionals are incorporating herbal remedies into their practices—but serious mental disorders require immediate medical attention. Moreover, some of the herbs used to treat mental problems (as well as other conditions) can interact with the prescription medications used by conventional practitioners. Be sure to talk with your doctor before using any herbal remedy to treat a psychological issue.

Handling Stress

Stress is a natural part of life. Quite often, it's psychological stress that gets you out of bed in the morning or to the gym in the evening. It's what makes you perform well at the office or in the classroom and do basically everything that you need to survive. Unfortunately, too much stress—problems that go on too long or demand too many of your resources—can wreak havoc on your health. Chronic, unresolved stress has been linked to a host of diseases, including cardiovascular disease and cancer. It's also been tied to many mental disorders, such as depression.

Of course, facing a stressful event—even if it's a terribly stressful one, such as the death of a spouse—doesn't necessarily mean you'll develop a mental illness. But stress can definitely up your chances of problems like depression or anxiety disorders. Herbs can help you deal with all kinds of stress—both psychological and physical.

- **Ashwagandha** (*Withania somnifera*)
Ashwagandha is an Ayurvedic remedy for stress-related anxiety and insomnia. Studies show it inhibits the release of stress hormones and calms the central nervous system.

- **Lavender** (*Lavandula angustifolia*)
The essential oil of this fragrant plant has proven antianxiety properties when applied topically or inhaled. In laboratory tests, it performed as well as the drug Valium.

- **Ginkgo** (*Ginkgo biloba*)
Ginkgo is famous for its brain-boosting powers. In the lab, it's shown an ability to offset many effects of stress, such as memory deficits and depression.

- **Asian ginseng** (*Panax ginseng*)
Asian ginseng is one of the best-researched herbs around, and it has been used for centuries to help people manage stress. Recent research has shown it can protect the brain from the damage caused by chronic stress.

- **Lemon balm** (*Melissa officinalis*)
This herb relieves stress and induces relaxation. Research shows it can improve your mood, increase your alertness (and mental processing speeds), and produce a general feeling of well-being.

- **Schisandra** (*Schisandra chinensis*)
This herb balances your nervous and endocrine (hormone) systems and is particularly good at helping you manage psychological stress. Research shows it can increase your mental performance and adjust the levels of the stress hormone cortisol in your system.

- **Saint John's wort** (*Hypericum perforatum*)
This herb has been shown to alleviate the cognitive effects of stress, such as lapses in working memory, as well as the decreased physical performance and feelings of anxiety that stress can also produce.

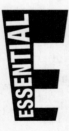

Stressful life events can trigger depression and can make a depressive episode more severe (and last longer). Research has shown that between 20 and 25 percent of people who experience a seriously stressful event become depressed. Studies of depressed people show that as many as 80 percent of them have experienced a major stress in the last six months.

Halting Anxiety

Anxiety disorders include several different conditions, such as generalized anxiety disorder (GAD), panic disorder, obsessive-compulsive disorder (OCD), post-traumatic stress disorder (PTSD), and phobias.

Anxiety disorders share a common feature: an uncontrollable and, in many cases unexplainable, fear or dread. In most cases, people with one type of anxiety disorder have another; anxiety disorders frequently accompany depression, as well.

Some anxiety disorders are treated with antidepressants like fluoxetine (Prozac), paroxetine (Paxil), and sertraline (Zoloft). Medications specifically made to treat anxiety include clonazepam (Klonopin), alprazolam (Xanax), and diazepam (Valium). Possible side effects include drowsiness, fatigue, loss of coordination, and mental confusion.

While serious anxiety disorders demand attention from a doctor (and may require the use of prescription drugs), many milder or episodic types of anxiety respond quite well to herbal remedies. For example:

- **Hops** (*Humulus lupulus*) — This is a traditional antianxiety treatment that helps relieve depression, as well. Hops also acts as a mild sedative.

- **Kava** (*Piper methysticum*) — Kava is the go-to herbal for anxiety, and has centuries of use (and research) behind it. The latest studies confirm its ability to relieve the symptoms of anxiety as well as the most frequently prescribed pharmaceuticals.

- **Passionflower** (*Passiflora incarnata*) — Recent research has shown that passionflower relieves anxiety symptoms as well as drugs, without the side effects. Other research shows it can relieve presurgery anxiety without unnecessary sedation.

- **Valerian** (*Valeriana officinalis*) — Valerian is a gentle sedative and mood stabilizer. Research shows that combining it with Saint John's wort (*Hypericum perforatum*) or kava (*Piper methysticum*) can relieve agitation and anxiety.

Depression and Other Mood Disorders

Depression is the best known of the illnesses classified as mood disorders, a group of conditions that includes major depression, dysthymic disorder (which is a type of chronic, mild depression), seasonal affective disorder (SAD), postpartum depression (PPD), and bipolar disorder.

Major or Minor

Everyone feels sad sometimes, but when those feelings linger or are so intense that they interfere with your daily functioning, they could be a sign of depression. Mood disorders generally involve feelings of persistent sadness, hopelessness, and apathy, but major depression, as its name implies, can create serious problems in an individual's personal and professional life and, in extreme cases, lead to suicide attempts.

ESSENTIAL

Exercise is a proven remedy for many psychological disorders, including anxiety, depression, ADHD, and age-related dementia. Research shows that a half-hour a day of exercise, three to five days a week, can significantly improve depression symptoms. Even shorter bouts of exercise —ten to fifteen minutes of physical activity—have been shown to boost your mood.

Depression often runs in families and typically begins before age thirty. It's much more common in women than in men. Both genetics and life experiences—nature as well as nurture—seem to play a role.

Depression is generally treated with antidepressants, which include old-school tricyclic antidepressants and monoamine oxidase inhibitors (MAOIs) as well as newer drugs called *selective serotonin reuptake inhibitors* (SSRIs). The SSRIs include fluoxetine (Prozac), paroxetine (Paxil), and sertraline (Zoloft). Over the past several years, drug companies have come up with a few more antidepressants, including venlafaxine (Effexor) and bupropion (Wellbutrin).

Side effects from antidepressants vary: Tricyclics and MAOIs have the worst, including constipation, bladder problems, blurred vision, and dizziness. SSRIs and the other new drugs can cause sexual side effects, headache, nausea, and agitation.

Bipolar Disorder

Bipolar disorder, also known as manic-depressive disorder, affects about 6 million Americans over the age of eighteen, or about 2.6 percent of the adult population. It encompasses two very serious mood problems: mania, which is a euphoric "high" that's often accompanied by reckless or even dangerous behavior, and depression.

Most often, antimanic (or mood-stabilizing) medications are used to treat bipolar disorder. The best known is lithium (Eskalith), which can cause fatigue, nausea, and tremors. Some patients are given an anticonvulsant, such as divalproex sodium (Depakote), which can cause headaches, double vision, dizziness, and anxiety.

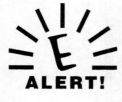
ALERT!

Although SSRIs are extremely popular (doctors wrote more than 31 million prescriptions in 2005), research shows that much of their perceived efficacy is due to the placebo effect and they actually work in less than half of the patients who try them. Some herbs and lifestyle factors (like exercise) have been shown to be just as effective.

While a serious or prolonged case of depression or bipolar disorder should be treated by a doctor, many people find that herbs can help relieve some symptoms. For example:

- **Boswellia** (*Boswellia serrata*)
  Boswellia produces a fragrant resin that is used as incense. New research has shown that it contains a psychoactive compound that relieves depression and anxiety.

- **Lemon balm** (*Melissa officinalis*)
  Lemon balm is used to treat depression and calm the highs of bipolar disorder.

- **Rhodiola** (*Rhodiola rosea*)
  Rhodiola has been proven effective against the symptoms of depression, both as an adjunct treatment (it was studied along with a tricyclic antidepressant drug) and on its own.

- **Saint John's wort** (*Hypericum perforatum*)
  This is a classic herbal remedy for depression—and one of the most researched herbs being used today. While not every study has shown a significant benefit, most experts agree that Saint John's wort can alleviate the symptoms of mild to moderate depression.

Attention Difficulties

Attention deficit hyperactivity disorder, or ADHD, is one of the most common mental disorders in children—and adults—today. The principal characteristics of ADHD are inattention, hyperactivity, and impulsivity. In most cases, ADHD shows up in preschool or early elementary school, but many people are not diagnosed until much later. It is estimated that between 3 and 5 percent of American children (and more than 4 percent of adults) have symptoms of ADHD.

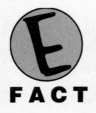

FACT

Between 1993 and 2003, the use of pharmaceutical ADHD treatments tripled (and spending on them increased ninefold, to roughly $2.4 billion), according to the National Institute of Mental Health. Doctors in the United States prescribe more than 80 percent of the world's ADHD medications.

ADHD is typically treated with stimulant medications, such as methylphenidate (Ritalin) and amphetamine mixed salts (Adderall). Other ADHD meds include the drug atomoxitine (Strattera), which is a nonstimulant. Side effects can include decreased appetite, insomnia, anxiety, and headache. Here are some herbal alternatives for attention difficulties:

- **American ginseng** (*Panax quinquefolius*) — Like its Asian cousin, *Panax ginseng*, this herb is a traditional remedy for taming psychological and physical stress and sharpening mental powers. Research shows that it can alleviate the symptoms of ADHD.
- **Ginkgo** (*Ginkgo biloba*) — Studies show that ginkgo can sharpen your mind, whether you're dealing with age-related decline or attention difficulties.
- **Flax** (*Linum usitatissimum*) — Flax contains alpha-linolenic acid (ALA), one member of a group of essential fatty acids called omega-3s, which have been shown to help with the symptoms of ADHD (and depression).
- **Maritime pine** (*Pinus pinaster*) — An extract from the bark of this French tree can reduce hyperactivity and increase attentiveness and concentration in people with ADHD.

Alcohol and Other Addictions

Addictions to alcohol, drugs, and other substances are an enormous problem in the United States and around the world, and are one of the biggest causes of preventable illness and death today.

Alcohol is a legal drug (for people twenty-one and older) in the United States, and most often it is a harmless part of our social lives. But excessive drinking can create enormous problems, including cirrhosis of the liver, heart disease, sexual dysfunction, and a cognitive disorder known as alcoholic dementia.

Marijuana is the most common illicit drug in the United States, although smoking it has been associated with short-term memory loss and other cognitive problems, elevated blood pressure and heart rate, and loss of motor skills.

Close behind marijuana are stimulants like cocaine and amphetamines, which can cause violent or erratic behavior, heart attack, seizure, or stroke. Opioids like heroin can damage the heart, lungs, and brain, and hallucinogens like ecstasy or LSD ("acid") cause hallucinations and flashbacks—and possibly death.

Addictive substances also include legal drugs: tranquilizers like alprazolam (Xanax) and diazepam (Valium), painkillers like oxycodone (OxyContin, Percocet), stimulants like methylphenidate (Ritalin), and sedatives like temazepam (Restoril) and triazolam (Halcion), all of which are highly addictive and can cause serious problems when abused.

ESSENTIAL

Rates of prescription and over-the-counter drug abuse are climbing. According to the U.S. Department of Health and Human Services, nonmedical use of prescription pain relievers was second only to marijuana among the types of illicit drug use in 2004. That same year, roughly 2 million people met the criteria for dependence or abuse involving a prescription drug.

Another legal yet addictive substance is the nicotine found in cigarettes and chewing tobacco. The U.S. Surgeon General has stated that the nicotine in tobacco products has addictive properties similar to heroin. According to government figures, nearly 58 percent of the nation's 61.6 million smokers—35.5 million people—meet the criteria for nicotine dependence.

Conventional medicine typically treats addictions with a combination of counseling and medications. Alcoholics are given drugs to help them reduce their dependence on alcohol, and people with addictions to drugs like heroin are given methadone, a synthetic opioid that helps ease them off their drug habit.

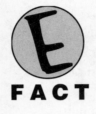

FACT

Researchers are investigating an experimental drug called *ibogaine*, which is a naturally occurring alkaloid chemical in the African iboga shrub (*Tabernanthe iboga*) that seems to turn off the brain messages associated with addictive behaviors and thus may be useful in treating drug, alcohol, and other addictions.

While serious cases of dependence require medical attention, many people have found some herbal remedies helpful in breaking the cycle of addiction, including:

- **Danshen** (*Salvia miltiorrhiza*)
Studies show that extracts inhibit alcohol absorption, reduce alcohol intake, delay the onset of "drinking behavior," and help prevent relapse drinking.

- **Kudzu** (*Pueraria lobata*)
Kudzu contains a chemical called diadzin that acts as an antidipsotropic (it causes a physical reaction when alcohol is consumed). Research shows it can reduce alcohol intake as well as the symptoms of withdrawal.

- **Passionflower** (*Passiflora incarnata*)
Passionflower reduces marijuana, nicotine, and alcohol withdrawal symptoms and helps relieve the sexual side effects of alcohol and nicotine abuse. It eliminates the addictive effects of drugs like morphine, and has been shown to be a useful adjunct therapy with the drug clonidine for opiate withdrawal.

- **Saint John's wort** (*Hypericum perforatum*)
In addition to its antidepressant qualities, Saint John's wort also suppresses alcohol consumption (and performs as well as the prescription drug Prozac in treating alcoholics).

CHAPTER 11

Improving Digestion

Around 400 B.C., Hippocrates—the Father of Medicine —reportedly gave us some words to live by: "Let food be thy medicine and medicine be thy food." The traditional schools of medicine in China, Europe, and India also stress digestion—and the use of nutritious and medicinal herbs—as a cornerstone of health. Herbal gastrointestinal aids and remedies work gently to support digestion and restore healthy functioning. Most produce no side effects and can be used safely in combination with other herbs as well as conventional medical treatments.

The Details of Digestion

Your digestive system converts everything you eat and drink into the fuel you need to function—and survive.

The digestive tract, also known as the gastrointestinal (GI) tract, transports and processes your meals, delivering essentials to your bloodstream and eliminating the rest. Its components include, in sequential order: mouth, esophagus, stomach, small intestine, and large intestine (colon). The system also includes the liver, which produces digestive juices, processes nutrients, and eliminates toxins.

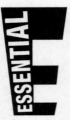

Your GI tract includes about thirty feet of hollow tubes—including your stomach, which holds less than a quarter-cup when empty and more than eight cups after a big buffet, and your small intestine, which contains millions of tiny villi that collectively make your intestinal surface area about 200 times bigger than that of your skin.

First, you chew your food and swallow it, propelling it into your esophagus. It's passed along through a series of involuntary smooth muscle movements into the stomach, where it's churned together with digestive juices and sent into the small intestine. Once there, it's combined with other juices, some from the intestine and others from the liver and pancreas.

In the small intestine, essential nutrients are absorbed into the bloodstream, and what's left—now considered waste—moves into the large intestine, where much of the remaining fluid is removed. It's then sent to the rectum, where it's eliminated.

Acid Indigestion and Heartburn

Acid indigestion, or *dyspepsia*, is a type of chronic or recurrent discomfort in the upper abdomen that's often accompanied by gas, bloating, and heartburn (a painful, burning sensation in your throat or chest).

Heartburn is the most common symptom of gastroesophageal reflux (GER), also known as *acid reflux*, a condition in which stomach acid backs up into your esophagus. Recurrent acid reflux is called *gastroesophageal reflux disease*, or GERD.

ALERT!

Heartburn and acid reflux, two of the most common digestive issues in the United States, can be triggered by many pharmaceuticals, including cardiac medications and drugs used to treat osteoporosis, insomnia, and anxiety. Both prescription and nonprescription pain medications have also been implicated, as have some oral contraceptives.

Heartburn and acid indigestion often run in families, but they can also be caused by lifestyle factors (smoking, obesity, drinking alcohol or caffeinated drinks, and eating foods that are very acidic or fatty). And while heartburn is most often only an annoyance, it can lead to more serious problems, including ulcers and precancerous cell changes.

Chronic heartburn can also be a symptom of serious conditions, including erosion of the esophagus and cancer.

Conventional Treatments

Dyspepsia, heartburn, acid reflux, and GERD are typically treated with these drugs:

- **Antacids.** Over-the-counter (OTC) remedies like sodium bicarbonate (Alka-Seltzer) neutralize acid and provide rapid heartburn relief; antacids can cause side effects like headaches, nausea, constipation, and diarrhea.
- **Acid Blockers.** Acid blockers like famotidine (Pepcid) and ranitidine (Zantac) reduce the amount of acid your stomach makes. They also can cause headaches, nausea, constipation, and other problems.
- **Bismuth Subsalicylate.** Bismuth subsalicylate (Pepto-Bismol, Kaopectate) balances the fluids in your GI tract. It can cause reactions in people who are allergic to aspirin and other salicylates and can make an ulcer or other bleeding problem worse. It can also interact with other drugs (including those prescribed to treat heart disease,

arthritis, and diabetes, as well as nonprescription pain relievers and cold medicines).

- **Proton Pump Inhibitors (PPIs).** People with GERD are often prescribed drugs called *proton pump inhibitors*, or PPIs, which stop your body's production of gastric acid. They include omeprazole (Prilosec), lansoprazole (Prevacid), and esomeprazole (Nexium). Prilosec OTC is a nonprescription option. Nearly 40 percent of the people who take them daily still experience symptoms—and must use additional drugs. PPIs can also cause abdominal pain and headaches, and they've been linked with increased risk of infection and pneumonia.

Herbal Answers

Many herbs have a long history of use in treating dyspepsia and reflux, including:

• **Artichoke** (*Cynara cardunculus, C. scolymus*)	Artichoke leaf extracts have been shown to significantly reduce dyspepsia symptoms, including heartburn and nausea.
• **Chamomile** (*Matricaria recutita*)	Chamomile is a traditional remedy for all kinds of GI problems, and research shows it can relieve spasms and reduce inflammation in gastrointestinal tissues.
• **Turmeric** (*Curcuma longa*)	This is a classic Ayurvedic remedy for digestive disorders—and studies show it can reduce the release of acid in the stomach.

Ulcers

An ulcer is an open sore caused by infection, poor circulation, or disease (people with diabetes often develop ulcers on their lower extremities). Within the digestive system, ulcers can occur in the esophagus, stomach, and small intestine; other ulcers can appear in the colon. Ulcers in the GI tract are generally known as peptic ulcers (peptin is an enzyme produced in the stomach).

While the classic image of someone with an ulcer is a red-faced, stressed-out, middle-aged man eating a spicy meal and washing it down with a stiff drink, scientists now know that ulcers aren't caused by stress, foods, or alcohol. Ulcers can strike anyone—about one in ten people will develop one at some point—and are almost always caused by *Helicobacter pylori* bacteria, which thrive in a highly acidic environment (as many as 80 percent of peptic ulcers are caused by *H. pylori* infection).

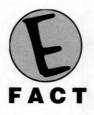
FACT

The GI system's natural defenses include microbes, known as gut flora, which can get a boost from probiotics (things that contain beneficial bacteria) or prebiotics (things that foster their growth). Many plants—including almonds (*Prunus dulcis*), garlic (*Allium sativum*), oats (*Avena sativa*), and wheat (*Triticum aestivum*)—contain prebiotics, which also might help prevent infections (including foodborne illness), ulcers, and cancer.

Symptoms of a peptic ulcer include abdominal pain (a gnawing or burning pain that comes on two or three hours after a meal or in the middle of the night) and bloating. Having a history of heartburn and GERD makes you more susceptible, as does taking certain pharmaceuticals, including NSAIDs and glucorticoids, which are steroids used to treat inflammation.

Treatment Options

If you've got a peptic ulcer, see your doctor right away. Left untreated, ulcers can cause potentially life-threatening internal bleeding. Conventional medicine generally treats peptic ulcers with antibiotics to kill the *H. pylori* infection (if it's present) and suppress stomach acid production. The drugs used to accomplish that are acid blockers and PPIs (see above).

Herbal remedies, which can be used in conjunction with conventional treatment, include these:

- **Aloe** (*Aloe vera*) Studies show that oral doses of aloe gel kill ulcer-causing bacteria, reduce inflammation, and promote healing of GI tissues.
- **Chamomile** (*Matricaria recutita*) This herb is famous for its soothing effects on the digestive tract. But it also has a tough side: Studies show it's lethal against ulcer-causing *H. Pylori* bacteria.

- **Gotu kola**
  (*Centella asiatica*)

  This Ayurvedic herb is valued for its wound-healing abilities. Extracts have been shown effective in treating peptic ulcers and helping to protect the stomach and GI tissues against them.

- **Marshmallow**
  (*Althaea officinalis*)

  Marshmallow leaves are a traditional European and Asian remedy for all sorts of GI inflammation, including peptic ulcers. Marshmallow contains polysaccharides, which form a gelatinous layer that helps promote healing.

- **Neem**
  (*Azadirachta indica*)

  This is a classic digestive and immunity-enhancing herb in Ayurvedic medicine, and modern research shows it can inhibit acid production and promote ulcer healing in the stomach.

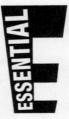

Because of their complex chemical structure, many herbs used traditionally to treat digestive and gastrointestinal problems actually address several problems at once. For example, licorice (*Glycyrrhiza glabra*) is a soothing demulcent, pain-killing analgesic, and antibacterial that can relieve the pain of ulcers, speed their healing, and prevent their return.

Gas and Flatulence

Everyone has gas—most of us generate between one and four pints a day (and pass some of it at least fourteen times). Gas is a natural by-product of the digestion process, and only causes problems when it's produced in excess.

The gas in your intestinal tract comes from two places: the air you swallow and the bacteria in your large intestine, which create gas as they break down the food that's passing through.

Some people have trouble digesting certain foods, and their bodies send partially digested food into the large intestine, where the bacteria produce extra gas as they "eat" it. For example, lactose, a sugar found in dairy products, can cause serious gas in people who don't produce enough of the lactose-digesting enzyme lactase. Other people are sensitive to artificial sweeteners like sorbitol and mannitol, which are used in sugar-free gum and other "diet" foods. Overuse of antibiotics or laxatives can also cause problematic gas.

Aside from the social embarrassment, gas can cause abdominal pain when it gets out of hand. Frequent or severe episodes warrant a visit to the doctor, as they can be the sign of a more serious problem.

Herbal Remedies

Herbal remedies for gas include:

- **Alfalfa** (*Medicago sativa*) — Alfalfa contains chlorophyll, which is the green ingredient in many herbs and some types of algae. Taking supplemental chlorophyll—and its derivative, chlorophyllin—has been shown to reduce gas (and its odor).
- **Caraway** (*Carum carvi*) — Caraway contains carminative (antigas) and antispasmodic constituents. Research shows that it can relieve gas and stomach upset.
- **Fennel** (*Foeniculum vulgare*) — A classic digestive aid throughout the Mediterranean, fennel seeds and extracts can relax the smooth muscles in the GI tract and expel gas.

Constipation

Constipation is defined as having infrequent or difficult bowel movements or passing hard or dry stools. "Infrequent" generally means fewer than three in a week, although some people regularly have two or three a day and others can go two or three days without one.

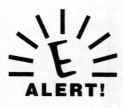
ALERT!

People who frequently use conventional chemical laxatives are prone to lazy bowel syndrome, a condition in which the digestive system has essentially become addicted to the drugs—and can't function properly without them. Overuse of laxatives can also damage your GI tract and interfere with your body's ability to absorb the nutrients in your food.

Constipation is most often tied to intestinal slowdown, in which the undigested food is moving too slowly through the large intestine. This can be caused by diet (inadequate fluid or fiber intake) as well as lifestyle factors like physical inactivity. Stress and traveling can trigger it, as can many prescription drugs. Pregnant women and people over sixty-five, especially those with physical limitations, are more susceptible.

Most of the time, you can resolve a case of constipation with a few tweaks to your diet or a dose or two of a laxative (either conventional or herbal). But if your condition persists or you experience other symptoms, see your doctor. Unresolved constipation can lead to complications like hemorrhoids or anal tears (called *abrasions* or *fissures*). In extreme cases, you could develop impaction, in which a mass of stool obstructs the colon or rectum. Constipation can also by a symptom of a more serious condition (see below).

Treatment Options

In conventional medicine, constipation is generally treated with laxatives, which fall into one of three categories:

- **Stool softeners** include mineral oil and medications containing docusate (Colace) or magnesium hydroxide (Philip's Milk of Magnesia), plus suppositories made with glycerine (Fleet Glycerin Suppositories).
- **Bulk-forming laxatives** create a more solid mass to keep things moving smoothly; they include methylcellulose (Citrucel, Docucal) and psyllium (Metamucil). Stool softeners and bulk-forming laxatives are generally free of side effects, but can cause abdominal pain and diarrhea in some people.
- **Stimulant (chemical) laxatives** trigger movement in the smooth muscles and induce secretion of fluids from the mucous membranes in the large intestine. They include polyethylene glycol (MiraLAX) and bisacodyl (Dulcolax, Correctol). Stimulant laxatives can cause cramping, lightheadedness, diarrhea, and rebound constipation.

Herbalism has its own constipation cures:

- **Flax**
  (*Linum usitatissimum*)

  Flaxseed is high in fiber (both the soluble and insoluble kind) and mucilage, which is a goopy substance known for its ability to sooth mucous membranes. Flaxseed works as an effective (and side effect-free) constipation remedy.

- **Fenugreek**
  (*Trigonella foenum-graecum*)

  Fenugreek also contains lots of fiber, including pectin, a type of insoluble fiber that's gelatinous when saturated with water (it's the ingredient in jelly that makes it gel).

- **Olive** (*Olea europa*) Olive oil acts as a gentle stool softener and laxative.
- **Psyllium** Both the blond and black varieties are tried-and-true constipation rem-
  (*Plantago ovata,* edies (*P. ovata* is the key ingredient in Metamucil). Research shows that
  P. psyllium) psyllium is as effective as many harsh chemical laxatives.

Diarrhea

Like constipation, diarrhea is something everyone has experienced: loose, watery, voluminous stools, accompanied by abdominal cramping, and frequent trips to the bathroom. Diarrhea is usually acute, lasting only a few days, but in some cases can become chronic, lasting more than a few weeks and possibly signifying a more serious condition. Persistent diarrhea can also lead to dehydration and loss of important minerals (such as salt).

When your digestive system is running smoothly, the food you've consumed travels through the GI tract as a liquid, until it hits the colon, where most of the liquid is absorbed (leaving behind a semi-solid waste). But if something happens to make the food pass too quickly through the colon (or to hinder the colon's ability to remove the liquid), you'll have watery bowel movements.

Acute diarrhea caused by infection is called *gastroenteritis*, which quite often is a type of foodborne illness (a.k.a. "food poisoning") that can usually be traced to a virus. It can also be caused by some diseases (including AIDS), exposure to toxins, and by taking certain medications—most often antibiotics, which destroy both beneficial and pathogenic bacteria in your digestive tract and can set the stage for infection. Blood pressure drugs and antacid medications containing magnesium can also trigger diarrhea.

Many people have food intolerances and sensitivities that bring on an acute bout of diarrhea whenever the offending food is consumed. Some of the most common examples are lactose (in milk and other dairy products), fructose (a type of sugar), and artificial sweeteners.

Chronic diarrhea, on the other hand, can be a sign of a serious condition. See a doctor if your diarrhea lasts longer than three days or if you become dehydrated (you're feeling lightheaded and are passing dark urine), are running a fever that's higher than 102°F, have bloody or black stools, or are in severe pain.

Treatment Options

Conventional medical practitioners typically recommend OTC antidiarrheal medications such as loperamide (Imodium) and bismuth subsalicylate (Kaopectate, Pepto-Bismol). Loperamide slows the transit of fluids through your GI tract, and bismuth subsalicylate balances the fluids in your intestinal tract. If your diarrhea is being caused by an infection, a doctor might prescribe antibiotics as well.

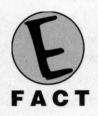

FACT

Pectin, a type of water-soluble fiber found in many fruits, vegetables, and herbs, can be used as a stand-alone treatment for diarrhea (it seems to increase the absorption of salt and water in the GI tract). To get it as nature intended, eat lots of apples (*Malus domestica*).

Loperamide can cause constipation and cramping. Bismuth subsalicylate can interact with other drugs and turn your tongue (and stools) temporarily black. Here are some herbal alternatives:

- **Barberry** (*Berberis vulgaris*)

  Barberry is a traditional herbal remedy for diarrhea and other digestive problems. It contains a chemical called berberine, which has proven antispasmodic, antimicrobial, and anti-inflammatory power.

- **Cinnamon** (*Cinnámomum verum, C. aromaticum*)

  Cinnamon can be used to treat diarrhea and other types of GI distress. It contains chemicals and essential oils that have been proven to relieve diarrhea, gas, and bloating.

- **Ginger** (*Zingiber officinale*)

  This is a classic remedy for diarrhea that's accompanied by nausea. In the lab, it has demonstrated anticramping properties—and the ability to kill foodborne *Salmonella* bacteria.

- **Juniper** (*Juniperus communis*)

  A traditional Native American remedy for all sorts of digestive ills, including stomachaches and diarrhea, juniper contains several chemicals with antidiarrheal and antimicrobial properties.

- **Psyllium** (*Plantago ovata, P. psyllium*)

  Psyllium, which is typically used to treat constipation (it works as a bulk-forming laxative), also fights diarrhea. Research shows it can be as effective as the drug loperamide.

- **Sangre de grado**   Research shows that sap of this South American tree can be effective
  (*Croton lechleri*)   against diarrhea caused by many types of infection.
- **Tea**   Tea contains tannins and other polyphenols, which have been shown to
  (*Camellia sinensis*)   relieve diarrhea as well as the drug loperamide.

Nausea and Vomiting

Nausea—defined as an upset stomach accompanied by the urge to vomit—can be a symptom of many conditions, some decidedly more worrisome than others. Vomiting can by a symptom of a serious problem like poisoning, head injury or brain tumor, infection (such as hepatitis), or another disease or condition (such as appendicitis, kidney failure, gallstones, or an ulcer).

Less scary causes include migraine headaches, pregnancy (morning sickness), and certain drugs. Many people become nauseated when they're in a moving vehicle (motion sickness); most of us feel nauseated when we've had too much to drink.

Treatment Options

Most cases of nausea are self-limiting: When you get out of the moving car, metabolize the alcohol in your system, or deliver the baby, the nausea will go away. However, if you think you've got food poisoning (or another type of poisoning), if you're experiencing severe abdominal pain or other pains (like a headache or stiff neck), are vomiting blood, or have been sick to your stomach for more than twenty-four hours, you should see a doctor right away.

Conventional medicine typically treats nausea and vomiting with anti-emetic (antinausea) drugs. Motion sickness is treated prophylactically with antihistamines—OTC drugs like meclizine (Bonine), dimenhydrinate (Dramamine), or prescription drugs like scopolamine (Transderm Scop). If you're already vomiting, you might take bismuth subsalicylate (Pepto-Bismol); see above. Antihistamines can cause drowsiness and, less often, headache, diarrhea or constipation, and irregular heartbeat; scopolamine can cause vision problems, dry mouth, and drowsiness. Here are some herbal alternatives:

- **American ginseng**
  (*Panax quinquefolius*)

  American ginseng is known for its antiemetic properties. In the lab, it's shown the ability to prevent nausea and vomiting before they start.

- **Ginger**
  (*Zingiber officinale*)

  Ginger can fight almost any type of nausea you can think of, including morning sickness, postoperative nausea, motion sickness, migraine-related nausea, and nausea caused by chemotherapy.

- **Lavender**
  (*Lavandula angustifolia*)

  Lavender is a traditional remedy for stomach upset, nausea, and vomiting (it contains camphor, a chemical with known antiemetic properties). The scent of lavender can also quell the queasies.

Food Intolerances

Food intolerances are much more common than allergies, affecting about 10 percent of all Americans, and are the sign of a problem in the digestive system. You're intolerant if a certain food irritates your stomach or intestines or if your body can't digest it properly. The most common type is lactose intolerance, which occurs in people who lack the enzyme lactase. Other intolerances occur in people who are sensitive to a certain chemical: Food dyes, monosodium glutamate (or MSG, which is a flavor enhancer often used by Chinese restaurants), and sulfites (which occur naturally but are also added to foods to inhibit mold) are common culprits.

ESSENTIAL

Food allergies can be triggered by a tiny amount of food—even residuals left over in a manufacturing facility—and occur every time you eat it, so experts advise people with food allergies to swear off that food completely. But food intolerances are often dose related, meaning you won't experience any symptoms unless you eat a lot of the food.

Food intolerance can produce nausea, diarrhea, cramping, gas and bloating, headaches, and irritability or nervousness. Here are some herbal remedies:

- **Ginger**
  (*Zingiber officinale*)

  Ginger is a proven stomach settler that also appears to have an antihistamine-like effect against food allergies.

- **Peppermint**
  (*Mentha x piperita*)

  Peppermint is a classic stomach soother that appears to "deactivate" the inflammatory response in laboratory tests. Research shows it can relieve dyspepsia, bloating, and cramping.

- **Rooibos**
  (*Aspalathus linearis*)

  Rooibos tea, also known as red bush tea, is a South African remedy for nausea and vomiting that also quells the allergic response.

Chronic Digestive Disorders

Sometimes, things like diarrhea, constipation, and vomiting are symptoms of more serious digestive disorders, such as irritable bowel syndrome or inflammatory bowel disease. These are known as "functional" bowel disorders because they are related to bowel functioning, not anatomical or structural problems.

Irritable Bowel Syndrome

Irritable bowel syndrome (IBS), also known as spastic colon, is a condition of unknown origin with no known cure. Symptoms are abdominal pain and either constipation or diarrhea (in most people, one is predominant, but many people alternate between the two); some patients also experience dyspepsia, nausea, and bloating.

IBS is treated in conventional medicine with antispasmodic drugs such as dicyclomine (Bentyl), which can cause blurred vision, dizziness, nausea, and weakness. Acid-reducing, antidiarrheal, and/or laxative drugs are also used (see above).

People with IBS can treat their symptoms with the herbal remedies discussed above, along with these:

- **Agrimony**
  (*Agrimonia eupatoria*)

  This herb contains tannins, which are astringent, making it useful for people with diarrhea-predominant IBS.

- **Artichoke**
  (*Cynara cardunculus,*
  C. scolymus)

  Artichoke extracts have been shown to help people with chronic digestive complaints, including IBS-related constipation and pain.

- **Peppermint**
  (*Mentha x piperita*)

  Peppermint leaves contain antispasmodic chemicals that can help relax the muscles in your GI tract and ease the gas and diarrhea caused by IBS.

Inflammatory Bowel Disease

Inflammatory bowel disease, or IBD, is much less common than IBS, affecting about 1 million Americans. IBD is immune-mediated, meaning it involves an exaggerated immune response to certain triggers and appears to have genetic and environmental causes. Some experts categorize it as an autoimmune disease.

There are two different forms of IBD: Crohn's disease and ulcerative colitis. Both are characterized by inflammation, abdominal pain, weight loss, and diarrhea. People with ulcerative colitis can also experience fever and blood in the stool. Crohn's disease usually involves the small intestine, but it can affect any part of the GI tract. Ulcerative colitis usually involves just the colon. IBD symptoms usually follow in a pattern of relapse and remission, and patients can go for years without symptoms, then have an attack that lasts from several weeks to several months.

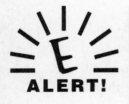

ALERT!

If you've got inflammatory bowel disease, avoid taking herbs with immune-enhancing effects, such as barberry (*Berberis vulgaris*), echinacea (*Echinacea purpurea*), and goldenseal (*Hydrastis canadensis*). Some experts think that the effects of these products might actually make IBD worse.

Conventional doctors generally treat IBD with antispasmodic drugs like Bentyl; anti-inflammatories such as sulfasalazine (Azulfidine) or a 5-ASA agent (Dipentum), which can cause nausea, heartburn, diarrhea, and headaches; or corticosteroids (see Chapter 8). Herbal remedies for diarrhea (see above) can be helpful, along with the following:

- **Boswellia** (*Boswellia serrata*) — Boswellia, a.k.a. Indian frankincense, contains natural anti-inflammatories. Preliminary research suggests that it can be effective against both Crohn's disease and ulcerative colitis.
- **Evening primrose** (*Oenothera biennis*) — Evening primrose oil contains gamma-linolenic acid (GLA) and linoleic acid, omega-6 fatty acids with proven anti-inflammatory effects.
- **Pineapple** (*Ananas comosus*) — An enzyme from pineapples called bromelain is used to promote proper digestion. Research shows it may be helpful in treating ulcerative colitis and the diarrhea that comes with it.

CHAPTER 12

Strengthening Immunity

Herbs have been used for centuries to support immune function and, when needed, to kick it into overdrive to beat an infection or disease. And while conventional medicine has traditionally focused its immune-system strategies on curing infections, herbalism has centered on the belief that supporting and nourishing the immune system will result in fewer and less severe infections—and better health overall. Happily, conventional practitioners are increasingly supportive of this notion, and research consistently proves the immune-boosting power of herbs.

Immunity and the Immune Response

It all starts here, with your immune response: the way your body recognizes and defends itself against bacteria, viruses, and any other foreign and potentially harmful substances. You won't stay healthy—or alive—for long if your immune system isn't working properly.

Your immune system is a layered series of defenses, starting with simple physical barriers (like your skin and mucous membranes) and finishing with a sophisticated system of chemical messengers and cellular warriors, designed to fend off attack from all kinds of disease-causing agents.

The immune system works by recognizing antigens and producing specific antibodies to destroy them. An antigen is any substance that is perceived by your body as a threat—and therefore causes your immune system to produce antibodies against it. Antigens can be foreign substances, such as bacteria, viruses, or chemicals, but they also can be formed within your body (examples might be cancer cells or the toxins created by invading bacteria).

The nemesis of any antigen is its antibody. Antibodies are a type of protein custom-made by the immune system to fight specific antigens. Each is unique and defends the body against only one type of antigen.

ESSENTIAL

Many chronic conditions, including diabetes, cancer, and liver disease, can reduce your body's resistance to germs, slow the healing of wounds, and set the stage for infection. So can poor nutrition, certain medications (like steroids), and anything that inhibits circulation and the flow of oxygen in your body, such as hypertension, heart disease, and smoking.

White blood cells, or leukocytes, seek out and destroy invading substances. One type of leukocytes are lymphocytes, which come in two varieties: B cells and T cells. B cells produce antibodies, and T cells attack antigens directly (they also help control the immune response).

Other chemicals include eicosanoids and cytokines, which are released by injured or infected cells and attract leukocytes and other immune cells to the scene to kill off the pathogens.

Your immune system also includes several structures—the lymph nodes, thymus, spleen, and marrow in the long bones in your arms and legs—that produce and store leukocytes.

Everyone has a few kinds of immunity, including:

- **Innate** (or nonspecific) immunity is your first line of defense, a set of built-in barriers that keep harmful substances out of your system. Examples include your skin, your cough reflex, and germ-fighting fluids like mucus, tears, and stomach acid.
- **Acquired** (or adaptive) immunity, also known as specific immunity, is created as you're exposed to various antigens and your body develops defenses to protect you against them. Your system "learns" to recognize and attack antigens and develops immunity to certain infections.

Immune Function and Disease

Over the course of your lifetime, your immune system will face a multitude of challenges—from external pathogens as well as your body's own tissues and processes. An infection occurs when bacteria or other microbes get into your body and begin to multiply. The situation officially turns into a disease when the infection does damage to the cells and tissues and creates symptoms of illness. Illness can also occur when your immune system is pushed off course by problems known as immune deficiency disorders, or *immunodeficiencies.*

When it comes to human health, infectious agents can be broken into four categories: parasites, bacteria, viruses, and fungi.

- Infectious parasites include the protozoa, or single-celled organisms, that cause malaria and a few types of foodborne illness. (Other protozoa, such as plankton, are harmless.)
- Bacteria are tiny, single-celled creatures that can live on nonliving surfaces (such as countertops and stair railings) as well as on (or in) a living host.

- Viruses are tiny microbes that contain one or two molecules of genetic material. They can't live on their own but instead must "hijack" living cells in order to survive and multiply.
- Fungi are actually primitive plants (they include mushrooms, molds, and yeasts).

In healthy people, the immune system is ready and able to meet most of the challenges it will face. You'll encounter pathogens and, if they're strong or plentiful enough, you'll develop an infection, which your body will eventually defeat, and you'll go on to fight another day.

However, in people with compromised immunity, even the smallest threat—or things that aren't threatening at all, such as allergens or the body's own cells—can create serious, potentially fatal problems.

ALERT!

Many herbs and supplements are known as "immune-stimulating" agents, but not every immune system needs stimulating: If you've got allergies, asthma, or an autoimmune disorder, you've got an overactive immune system. Thus, you need something that's "immune-modulating" to help regulate your body's immune response (and turn it down, if necessary).

Herbs: Your Immune System's Best Friend

Herbal medicine has a centuries-old tradition of nurturing immune function —of keeping people healthy by treating them before they get sick—with an array of immunity-modulating and immunity-boosting plants.

One of the guiding principles of herbal medicine is the support of immune functioning through herbs known as adaptogens or tonics (see Chapter 2). Adaptogenic herbs help your body deal with the ill effects of stress—which can be caused by many things, including trauma, injury, or infection—without getting sick. Tonics are typically used to shore up a system that needs "toning" or "tonifying" (meaning it's failing or just performing below par).

Several herbs have demonstrated a direct effect on the immune system. Some, like barberry (*Berberis vulgaris*), echinacea (*Echinacea purpurea*), and goldenseal (*Hydrastis canadensis*), contain high concentrations of chemicals that increase immune system activity and thus are considered *immunostimulants.*

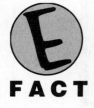

FACT

Exercise is a proven immunity booster. It flushes bacteria and other pathogens from the respiratory and urinary tracts (and skin, via sweat), increases circulation of antibodies and white blood cells, and slows the release of the stress-related hormones that can contribute to disease. Exercise even raises your body temperature, which acts like a fever to kill off infectious microbes.

Other herbs contain constituents that modulate the immune response, increasing immune activity when it's called for (i.e., when an infection is looming) and turning it down when necessary (in the case of allergies or autoimmune disorders). These are called *immunomodulators*, and they include astragalus (*Astragalus membranaceus*), Asian ginseng (*Panax ginseng*), licorice (*Glycyrrhiza glabra*), and reishi (*Ganoderma lucidum*); many of the herbs known as adaptogens are considered immunomodulators.

Sneezes, Sniffles, and Sore Throats

Upper respiratory infections are among the most common illnesses in the United States. They're highly contagious and are spread by both airborne particles and particles passed through physical contact (touching an infected person or an object he's touched). Colds or flu can precipitate other problems, such as bronchitis or sinusitis (inflammation in the bronchial passages or sinuses).

Colds are caused by viruses—experts have identified at least 200 different kinds—most of which cause sneezing, scratchy throat, and runny nose.

Influenza, or the flu, is a more severe upper respiratory infection caused by the influenza virus (there are three types, commonly known as A, B, and C, of which A and B are the most serious). Flu symptoms are more intense than those of a cold and typically include fever and muscle aches.

Strep throat is caused, as you might have guessed, by *Streptococcus* (strep) bacteria. It's characterized by sudden and acute throat pain and sometimes fever, headache, nausea, and vomiting. In most cases, your throat will be bright red and the lymph nodes in your neck will be swollen and tender.

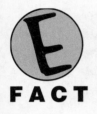

FACT

Hand washing is the best way to avoid catching many kinds of infections (cold and flu viruses can live up to three hours on your skin and just as long on hard surfaces like telephones and stair railings). Try using soap or liquid cleanser made with rosemary (*Rosmarinus officinalis*): It has proven antiviral and antibacterial powers.

Treatment Options

Strep infections are always treated with antibiotics like penicillin. To relieve throat pain, most conventional doctors recommend over-the-counter (OTC) sprays or lozenges made with topical anesthetics like benzocaine, which can cause irritation or allergic reactions in some people.

To prevent the flu, experts recommend an annual flu shot (or Flumist, a nasal spray). Some doctors also prescribe antiviral drugs like zanamivir (Relenza) and oseltamivir (Tamiflu), which can prevent an infection or lessen its severity and duration if taken within forty-eight hours of onset. These drugs can produce side effects like abdominal pain, diarrhea, and nausea.

Most people treat colds and flu with OTC pain relievers, decongestants, antihistamines, and cough medicines. These drugs can cause a long list of side effects, including irregular heartbeat, drowsiness, and stomach pain (see Chapter 13). Here are some herbal options:

- **Andrographis** (*Andrographis paniculata*)

  Andrographis is used in Ayurvedic and Chinese medicine to treat upper respiratory tract infections (it's an antibacterial and antioxidant). Studies show that it can relieve the symptoms of sore throats and helps to prevent colds.

- **Astragalus** (*Astragalus membranaceus*)

  Astragalus is used in Traditional Chinese Medicine as a tonic for the immune system. Studies show that it's an antiviral, antibacterial, and immunomodulator that helps prevent infections.

- **Echinacea**
  (*Echinacea purpurea*)

  Echinacea is a powerful antiviral and immune system stimulant, and has been shown in several studies to reduce the severity and duration of cold and flu symptoms.

- **Elderberry**
  (*Sambucus nigra*)

  Elderberry has both antiviral and immune-boosting effects, making it a great remedy for colds and flu. Research shows it can fight several viruses at once—and improve your symptoms in just a few days.

- **Ginger**
  (*Zingiber officinale*)

  Ginger inhibits the bacteria and viruses responsible for upper respiratory infections and also relieves sore throats and the aches of the flu.

- **Isatis**
  (*Isatis tinctoria*)

  Constituents of this Chinese herb have antiviral, antibacterial, antifungal, analgesic, and antipyretic (fever reducing) activity.

Common Viral Infections

The most common viral infections in humans, by far, are colds and flu. But viruses can also cause infections and diseases ranging from mild (mononucleosis) to severe (dengue fever and AIDS).

Warts

Warts are small, generally harmless growths on the skin. Most often they're just ugly, but in some cases they can be problematic. Common warts appear most often on the hands; plantar warts are on the soles of the feet; genital warts are found in the pubic area and on the genitals. They're caused by human papillomavirus, or HPV, a version of which can lead to cervical cancer.

OTC wart medications containing concentrated salicylic acid (Compound W, Transversal PlantarPatch) are often recommended for warts (except those on the face or genitals). These products dissolve the wart over a period of weeks, but they're highly corrosive and can burn the surrounding skin if not applied carefully. Some doctors prescribe stronger medications or remove warts via surgery, cyrotherapy (freezing), or electrocautery (burning). Genital warts are often treated with topical applications of imiquimod (Aldara), an immunomodulating drug that can cause itching, burning, and other side effects.

Cold Sores

Cold sores, also known as oral herpes or fever blisters, are caused by a type of herpes simplex virus (a relative of the one that causes genital herpes; see below). This infection is highly contagious—and permanent (it can recur indefinitely). After the initial sore heals, the virus settles into a dormant state in your nerve cells, where it will remain until it's reactivated (often by stress, trauma, or excessive sun exposure).

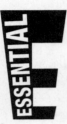

Many plants are natural antivirals. Green tea extracts can fight flu viruses and are also the key ingredient in sinecatechines (Veregen) ointment, a prescription drug that's approved by the FDA as a treatment for genital warts. Another genital wart drug, podophyllotoxin (Podofilox), is derived from two types of mayapple trees, *Podophyllum peltatum* and *P. hexandrum*.

Treatment Options

Conventional medicine treats viral infections with oral or topical prescription medications such as acyclovir (Zovirax) or penciclovir (Denavir), which suppress the virus. Acyclovir can cause side effects like diarrhea and vomiting (in the oral preparation) and burning and inflammation (in the topical form). Topical denavir can cause headache, skin reactions, and changes in your sense of smell or taste. These herbs offer another type of relief:

- **Echinacea** (*Echinacea purpurea*) Echinacea is a powerful weapon against viral infections. It's lethal to several pathogenic viruses, including the strain of herpes that causes cold sores, and can help boost your internal defenses as well.

- **Garlic** (*Allium sativum*) Garlic is a proven antiviral and can help fight infection both inside and out. Research shows that fresh garlic extracts can eradicate the viruses that cause herpes (as well as influenza and the common cold), and an isolated garlic compound has been shown effective against warts.

- **Isatis** (*Isatis tinctoria*) This Chinese herb, taken in combination with astragalus (*Astragalus membranaceus*), accelerates the healing of cold sores and warts.

- **Lemon balm** (*Melissa officinalis*) Topical applications can reduce the size and severity of cold sores, shorten their healing time, and prevent the spread of the infection.

- **Licorice**
  (*Glycyrrhiza glabra*)

  Licorice root contains phytochemicals that have been proven effective against several types of infectious viruses, including those that cause cold sores.

- **Sage**
  (*Salvia officinalis,*
  S. lavandulaefolia)

  Applied topically, sage extracts can halt viral infections. Research shows that a combination of sage and rhubarb (*Rheum officinale, R. palmatum*) can heal cold sores as well as the prescription drug acyclovir.

Bacterial Infections

Bacteria are everywhere, and most of the time they're harmless (some are even beneficial to human health, such as the *Lactobacillus*, a.k.a. "friendly" bacteria, in yogurt). But whenever there's a break in the structural integrity of your skin—whether it's a burn, a superficial scrape, or a deep puncture—you're opening the door to bacteria. If enough of them get in to overpower your body's defenses, you'll have an infection.

Wounds

Although any wound is open to bacterial invasion, open wounds (ulcers), large or severe burns, and bites are the most likely to become infected. Signs of infection include acute pain (it hurts more than you think it should), pus, and swelling that extends past the immediate area and feels hot.

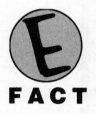

Many bacterial infections in humans can be traced to two kinds of bugs: *Staphylococcus* (staph) and *Streptococcus* (strep) bacteria. Staph infections typically involve the skin but can also affect the internal organs. Strep bacteria cause strep throat as well as several skin infections. Both are producing increasing numbers of drug-resistant strains.

Conventional treatment will depend on the severity of the infection. In many cases, you'll be given a prescription for oral antibiotics that are effective against the bacteria causing your infection. Oral antibiotics can contribute to the development of drug-resistant bacteria, and taking them long term can compromise your immunity.

Folliculitis

This inflammation of the hair follicles can occur anywhere there's hair. In most cases, the problem starts when the follicles are damaged by friction or abrasion (as in shaving), or blockage (wearing tight clothing), then invaded by *Staphylococcus* bacteria.

Conventional medicine typically treats folliculitis with antibacterial cleansers like triclosan (Dial Antibacterial Moisturizing Body Wash) or triclocarban (Safeguard Antibacterial Soap). These are serious chemicals—they're also used in industrial disinfectants—that have been linked to neurological and hormonal problems. You also may be given a prescription for an oral antibiotic (see above) or a topical antibiotic like mupirocin (Bactroban), which can cause burning, pain, and itching.

Other Skin Infections

Impetigo is a superficial skin infection caused by staph or strep bacteria. It produces small blisters or scabs that generally start on the face and may move to other parts of the body.

Cellulitis is an infection of the deep layers of the skin caused by bacteria—most often strep—that enter through a cut, burn, or other skin injury. Left untreated, it can spread to the lymph nodes and become life threatening. People who already have another type of infection or a chronic condition (like diabetes) that can impair circulation are most at risk of developing cellulitis.

Conventional Versus Herbal Solutions

Conventional medicine treats impetigo with prescription-strength topical antibiotics (see above); more serious cases might get a prescription for oral antibiotics. Cellulitis is treated with oral antibiotics (see above).

Many herbal remedies can be used alone or in conjunction with antibiotics to treat bacterial infections:

- **Barberry**
  (*Berberis vulgaris*)
  Barberry contains powerful antibacterial and anti-inflammatory chemicals that can inhibit bacteria from attaching to human cells. The same antibacterial chemicals are found in goldenseal (*Hydrastis canadensis*).

- **Cat's claw**
  (*Uncaria guianensis,
  U. tomentosa*)

  This traditional Peruvian remedy has proven antimicrobial effects—and can inhibit the activity of strep, staph, and other bacteria. It's also a proven anti-inflammatory and immunomodulator.

- **Gotu kola**
  (*Centella asiatica*)

  This herb is used in Ayurvedic medicine to foster all kinds of tissue repair. Recent research shows its ability to kick-start immune response, speed skin healing, and inhibit bacterial growth.

- **Saint John's wort**
  (*Hypericum
  perforatum*)

  Best known for its antidepressant capabilities, Saint John's wort is also a traditional remedy for skin problems caused by bacterial infection.

- **Witch hazel**
  (*Hamamelis
  virginiana*)

  Witch hazel bark is a classic treatment for itchy and inflamed skin (it's also astringent, so it helps dry up blisters). Recent research shows it can help halt staph infections (even the drug-resistant kind).

Fungal Infections

The world is full of molds, yeasts, and other types of fungi, most of which do more good than harm (think beer and penicillin). And most of the time, even pathogenic fungi can live in and on the body without any problem. But these organisms can cause infection if their numbers get out of control or if the body's immune system is suppressed.

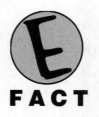

FACT

Ringworm has nothing to do with worms (even though its scientific name, *tinea*, means "growing worm" in Latin.) It got its moniker because a *tinea capitis* infection sometimes has a round shape, as if a worm were curled up under the skin. Ringworm is an infection of a type of fungi called *dermatophytes*, which may—or may not—line up in a ring-like formation.

Tinea Infections

Parasitic fungi called *dermatophytes* are responsible for the superficial skin infections commonly, if crudely, known as ringworm (*tinea capitis*), athlete's foot (*tinea pedis*), and jock itch (*tinea cruris*). A tinea infection usually isn't serious, but it can be itchy and uncomfortable; when it strikes the scalp, it can cause hair loss. Tinea-causing fungi thrive in warm, damp places, and are spread by direct contact: You can catch them by touching a person (or a pet) who's infected or from a damp surface, such as the shower in the health club.

Tinea infections can also occur around and under the nails—most often, the toenails—leaving them yellowed, thickened, and crumbling. This condition is called *tinea unguium*.

Candida Infections

Candida infections, called *candidiasis*, are caused by the yeast-like fungus *Candida albicans*. Vaginal candidiasis is characterized by sticky white or yellowish discharge, burning, and itching (see Chapter 3). Other *Candida* infections include oral thrush, which affects the mouth and throat, and skin infections like intertrigo (which occurs in skin folds) and some cases of diaper rash (see Chapter 6).

Conventional Treatments

Most tinea infections are treated with OTC topical antifungals such as clotrimazole (Mycelex, Lotrimin), or miconazole (Desenex, Monistat), which occasionally cause skin reactions. Scalp ringworm and toenail fungus are almost always treated with oral medications like itraconazole (Sporanox) or terbinafine (Lamisil), which can cause intestinal problems, rashes, and headaches. In cases of scalp ringworm, OTC dandruff shampoos that contain selenium sulfide (Selsun Blue) are sometimes recommended to prevent the spread of the fungi, but they can't eliminate it.

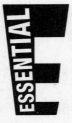

Newborns can actually be more resistant to infection than you'd think. Every baby is born with a set of built-in antibodies that were passed along from his mother, which creates what's known as passive immunity. By his first birthday, however, the child will have lost this protection—and his body will already have started making antibodies of its own.

Candidiasis is treated conventionally with OTC antifungal remedies such as miconazole (Monistat) and butoconazole (Mycelex), which can cause skin reactions and intestinal discomfort. Some doctors may also prescribe oral antifungals, such as fluconazole (Diflucan) or ketoconazole (Nizoral). Fluconazale can cause diarrhea and headaches; ketoconazole can cause nausea and abdominal pain.

Herbal Alternatives

Herbal remedies can be used in conjunction with these medicines, and include the following:

- **Camphor** (*Cinnamomum camphora*) — This natural fungicide can clear up a case of *tinea unguium* (research shows it's active against the most common fungal culprits).

- **Echinacea** (*Echinacea purpurea*) — This immune-boosting herb can help pharmaceuticals fight fungal infections even better than they could alone. Research shows that combining an oral echinacea preparation with a conventional antifungal cream can significantly reduce the rate of recurrent infections.

- **Garlic** (*Allium sativum*) — Fresh garlic extracts are lethal to tinea-causing fungi, and research using ajoene, an isolated garlic constituent, found that it cleared up athlete's foot, ringworm, and jock itch infections as well as the prescription drug terbinafine.

- **Lavender** (*Lavandula angustifolia*) — A natural anesthetic and anti-inflammatory, lavender oil is also an effective weapon against the *Candida albicans* fungus.

- **Pomegranate** (*Punica granatum*) — Pomegranate has proven fungicidal and wound-healing properties. Topically applied extracts of pomegranate peel, combined with gotu kola (*Centella asiatica*), have been shown to clear up oral candidiasis as well as pharmaceutical antifungals.

- **Tea tree** (*Melaleuca alternifolia*) — A traditional Aboriginal treatment for all types of skin inflammation, tea tree oil can also kill *Candida albicans* and other fungi.

Immunodeficiency Disorders

Immunodeficiency disorders—a class of conditions that includes primary (inherited) and secondary (acquired) disorders—can create a seemingly endless stream of infections that often lead to serious complications. For example, people with acquired immunodeficiency syndrome (AIDS) are prone to opportunistic infections, which are potentially life-threatening conditions that might not cause any problem in a healthy person. AIDS also makes infections harder to treat and creates more serious complications from run-of-the-mill infections like a cold or the flu.

Conventional medicine typically treats immunodeficiency disorders with drugs designed to prevent specific infections: antivirals like amantadine (Symmetrel) or acyclovir (Zovirax) or vaccines that protect against infections like the flu.

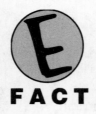

FACT

Immunodeficiency disorders can come from a prolonged illness (like cancer or diabetes) or infection (AIDS is caused by the HIV virus). Malnutrition can also trigger them—a shortfall of nutrients that puts you at less than 80 percent of your recommended weight can cause severe immune system impairment—as can immunity-suppressing treatments like chemotherapy and radiation.

Several herbs can also help support immune function to treat or prevent secondary infections (although experts warn people with immunity deficiencies to avoid immunostimulating herbs). Herbs can also treat the various symptoms of infection and relieve the side effects of conventional drug therapies. They include:

- **Amla** (*Emblica officinalis, Phyllanthus emblica*)

  Also known as amalaki, this Ayurvedic herb is an adaptogen, antioxidant, and antiviral; it's also a key ingredient in the Ayurvedic remedy known as triphala. Studies show it can speed the healing of infected wounds, inhibit the activity of HIV, and kill several types of infectious bacteria in HIV-infected patients.

- **Licorice** (*Glycyrrhiza glabra*)

  A staple in the pharmacies and pantries of China, Europe, and the Middle East, licorice has proven immunomodulating effects, which can help avert secondary infections.

- **Lemon balm** (*Melissa officinalis*)

  Lemon balm is a traditional remedy for viral infections, and extracts have shown specific activity against HIV. Peppermint (*Mentha x piperita*) and sage (*Salvia officinalis, S. lavandulaefolia*) have similar anti-HIV action.

- **Tea tree** (*Melaleuca alternifolia*)

  This herb is a potent antimicrobial, and research shows it can kill the *Candida* fungi that cause infections in immune-compromised people.

CHAPTER 13

The Herbal Medicine Cabinet

Most of the time, you're (thankfully) dealing with run-of-the-mill complaints and not dire emergencies or deadly diseases. But while problems like stomachaches and sunburns aren't life threatening, they do require remedies, and most people would rather avoid a middle-of-the-night trek to the drugstore by having the right medicine on hand. Conventional medicines are the standard in most American medicine cabinets, but many carry unwanted, even dangerous, side effects. Herbs offer a better solution.

Building a Better Medicine Chest

There are more than eighty categories of nonprescription, over-the-counter (OTC) drugs available in the United States today, treating everything from acne to warts. If you're like most people, you keep a supply of OTC remedies to treat the health concerns that you and your family face most often: headaches and head colds, diarrhea and indigestion, sleeplessness and sunburns.

But why stock your medicine cabinet (and body) full of synthetic medicines with unwanted side effects when there are herbal equivalents that can give you similar results with a more gentle approach? To build a better medicine chest, stock up on these herbal remedies.

Pain Relievers

OTC analgesics and anti-inflammatories certainly come in handy when you have a headache, sore muscles, or a hangover, but are they always the best choice? These herbs offer similar (if not better) pain relief than traditional OTC medications:

- **Arnica**
  (*Arnica montana*)

  In a recent study, topical arnica outperformed both topical ibuprofen and oral acetaminophen in relieving joint pain and stiffness. Arnica has also been proven effective at treating sore muscles and bruises.

- **Barberry**
  (*Berberis vulgaris*)

  Barberry works as both an internal and external painkiller. It's also an effective topical antimicrobial.

- **Cayenne**
  (*Capsicum annuum*)

  Applied to a sore spot, cayenne is a potent painkiller (its key constituent, capsaicin, is used in many OTC muscle and joint rubs and is approved by the FDA as a topical analgesic). Topical cayenne has also been shown to relieve and even prevent headaches.

- **Clove**
  (*Syzygium aromaticum*)

  Clove oil works as a topical pain reliever and anesthetic (and also fights bad breath and cavities, thanks to its antibacterial components). It's especially helpful after dental work, and research shows it fights pain as well as the OTC pharmaceutical benzocaine. Clove oil also soothes cold and canker sores and helps kill infectious microbes.

- **Cramp bark**
  (*Viburnum opulus*)

  An aptly named plant, cramp bark is a classic herbal remedy for muscle cramps (it's also a great headache remedy). Recent research shows it's also effective against spasmodic back pain.

- **Devil's claw** (*Harpagophytum procumbens*)

  Devil's claw has been used for generations in South Africa to treat pain and inflammation. Recent research has shown it's particularly effective against back pain.

- **Feverfew** (*Tanacetum parthenium*)

  Best known as a migraine remedy, feverfew is a staple of Western herbal medicine and a reliable remedy for all kinds of headaches (plus fevers and other kinds of inflammation).

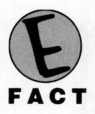

FACT

Tea tree oil (*Melaleuca alternifolia*) is a close as you'll get to a one-bottle medicine cabinet: It's got analgesic, anesthetic, antiseptic, antimicrobial, anti-inflammatory, deodorant, decongestant, and expectorant abilities. Research shows that topical tea tree oil can replace your acne medication, athlete's foot spray, mouthwash, deodorant, and cough medicine.

Better Cold and Flu Remedies

Instead of the conventional decongestants, antihistamines, and cough syrups, stock up on these botanicals:

- **Andrographis** (*Andrographis paniculata*)

  This Ayurvedic herb can significantly improve cold and sore throat symptoms; it also seems to prevent colds.

- **Astragalus** (*Astragalus membranaceus*)

  This herb is used in Traditional Chinese Medicine as an immunity-boosting tonic (it supports overall immune function and helps the body deal with the stress that can lead to infections and disease). Research shows that taking astragalus can help you avoid catching a cold.

- **Echinacea** (*Echinacea purpurea*)

  Echinacea has been studied extensively in recent years and proven to be an effective remedy for colds and other infections.

- **Elderberry** (*Sambucus nigra*)

  Elderberry is a classic European remedy for the flu (it has both antiviral and immune-boosting effects). Research shows that taking an elderberry extract can significantly improve flu symptoms in two to four days.

- **Isatis** (*Isatis tinctoria*)

  Constituents of this Chinese herb have antiviral, antibacterial, antifungal, analgesic, and antipyretic (fever reducing) activity. Isatis can both prevent and treat colds and flu.

- **Garlic**
  (*Allium sativum*)

  Garlic has antibacterial and antiviral properties and also seems to stimulate immunity, making it a good safety net against colds and flu. It's even shown effectiveness against antibiotic-resistant strains of oral strep bacteria.

- **Ginger**
  (*Zingiber officinale*)

  Ginger is a classic remedy for colds and flu (research shows it inhibits the bacteria and viruses responsible for upper respiratory infections); it's also an effective pain remedy. Ginger teas and syrups make a great stand-in for conventional cough and cold medicines.

- **Licorice**
  (*Glycyrrhiza glabra*)

  When it comes to fighting colds and flu, licorice qualifies as a one-herb wonder. It's used to soothe sore throats, quiet coughs, loosen chest congestion, clear nasal passages, and relieve pain.

- **Peppermint**
  (*Mentha x piperita*)

  Peppermint is the original source for menthol, which is used in many commercial chest rubs and other congestion-busting products. Inhaling the (diluted) essential oil or applying it to your skin can clear your head and chest.

- **Slippery elm**
  (*Ulmus rubra*)

  Slippery elm is a classic Native American sore throat remedy, thanks to its soothing demulcent properties.

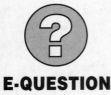

E-QUESTION

Can herbs help hangovers?
Research shows that taking extracts of red clover (*Trifolium pratense*) directly after drinking alcohol—or prickly pear (*Opuntia ficus-indica*) a few hours before drinking—can reduce your chance of getting a hangover by 50 percent. Cheers!

Tummy Treatments

Unlike conventional diarrhea, nausea, and constipation remedies, which attack only the symptoms of a particular problem, many herbs used to treat gastrointestinal problems actually help promote optimal digestion. Here are a few to keep on hand:

- **Artichoke**
  (*Cynara cardunculus,*
  C. scolymus)

  Artichoke is a classic (and proven) remedy for acid indigestion and heartburn, as well as the gastrointestinal pain, cramping, bloating, and flatulence of irritable bowel syndrome (IBS).

- **Fennel**
  (*Foeniculum vulgare*)

  Fennel relaxes the smooth muscles in the GI tract and helps eliminate gas and its odor. Chewing fennel seeds is a great breath freshener, too.

- **Flax**
  (*Linum usitatissimum*)

  Flaxseed is high in soluble and insoluble fiber (which fight constipation and speed elimination) and mucilage, which is soothing to irritated intestinal tissues. Both the seeds and oil are used to calm GI distress.

- **Ginger**
  (*Zingiber officinale*)

  Ginger is an effective and safe remedy for all kinds of nausea and vomiting, including motion sickness, morning sickness, postoperative nausea, migraine-related nausea, and nausea caused by chemotherapy.

- **Lavender**
  (*Lavandula angustifolia*)

  Lavender can be used internally to relieve stomach upset and dyspepsia (acid indigestion). It contains camphor, which is a carminative (it relieves gas) and antispasmodic (it relieves spasms in the gastrointestinal tract).

- **Peppermint**
  (*Mentha x piperita*)

  Peppermint is a traditional European remedy for stomach cramps, heartburn, and dyspepsia. A combination of peppermint and caraway (*Carum carvi*) has been shown to relieve the symptoms of chronic dyspepsia as well as prescription medicines.

- **Pineapple**
  (*Ananas comosus*)

  Pineapples contain the enzyme bromelain, which has protein-digesting abilities and can help promote proper digestion and relieve heartburn.

- **Psyllium**
  (*Plantago ovata*)

  Blond psyllium is used as bulk-forming agent to treat constipation (it's the key ingredient in the OTC drug Metamucil); psyllium is also an effective diarrhea remedy. Research shows that psyllium is as effective as harsh commercial laxatives in treating constipation and also works as well as the antidiarrheal drug loperamide.

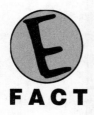

FACT

Many herbs used traditionally to spice up foods also posses stomach-soothing abilities. For example, both turmeric (*Curcuma longa*), the ingredient that gives curry its kick, and cardamom (*Elettaria cardamomum*), an aromatic spice used throughout India and Southeast Asia, can settle an upset stomach, relieve acid indigestion, and help heal and prevent ulcers.

Preventing Sunburns

Everybody knows that sunburns are bad: They cause wrinkles and old-before-its-time skin as well as cancer. Many herbs offer natural sun protection, some when applied directly to the skin, others when consumed as a food or drink—and others in both ways.

- **Coleus**
  (*Coleus forskohlii, Plectranthus barbatus*)

  Extracts of this Indian plant actually produce a "tan" without the accompanying skin damage. Coleus seems to stimulate production of melanin, the chemical that provides the skin's natural sun protection (people who tan easily or who have naturally dark skin are less susceptible to burning and skin cancer).

- **Grape**
  (*Vitis vinifera*)

  Grape skins are rich in antioxidants, nature's way of protecting the fruits from sunburn, and can convey the same benefits to human skin (grape seeds also contain them). You can apply grape extracts to your skin or consume them orally via grapes or wine.

- **Maca**
  (*Lepidium meyenii*)

  A native of the Peruvian Andes, maca developed a natural sunscreen to protect itself from all that high-altitude radiation. Research shows that topical maca extracts can also protect skin against UV damage.

- **Sesame**
  (*Sesamum indicum*)

  Used topically, sesame oil delivers natural sun protection.

- **Shea**
  (*Vitellaria paradoxa*)

  Also known as karite, shea nuts contain allantoin, a natural sunscreen (shea also contains skin-soothing moisturizers). Commercial products, usually sold as "shea butter," can add an extra dose of sun protection to your regular skin care routine.

- **Tomato** (*Lycopersicon esculentum*)

  Eating cooked tomatoes or tomato paste can make you less susceptible to sunburns and UV-related skin damage.

- **Spinach**
  (*Spinacia oleracea*)

  Spinach contains beta-carotene, which has been shown to reduce sunburn in fair-skinned people (one study combining beta-carotene supplements with vitamin E found a significant reduction in burns). Tossing spinach with other beta-carotene sources like beets (*Beta vulgaris*), carrots (*Daucus carota*), and watercress (*Nasturtium officinale*) can create the healthiest salad under the sun.

- **Tea**
  (*Camellia sinensis*)

  Green tea, which is rich in antioxidant polyphenols, can act as a natural sunscreen when applied to the skin (it's used in several commercial products). Studies show that drinking tea can also prevent sun damage.

The oils from coconuts (*Cocos nucifera*), sunflowers (*Helianthus annuus*), and olives (*Olea europaea*) also contain natural sunscreens.

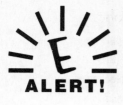

Your sunscreen is only as good as your application: The American Academy of Dermatology recommends about an ounce (what it takes to fill a shot glass) for the average adult, but studies show that most people use only about a quarter of that—and get about a quarter of the sun protection they think they're getting.

Beating Sleeplessness

Insomnia, the Latin term for "no sleep," is the inability to fall asleep—or stay asleep—and the problems related to it, such as waking up feeling tired. It's the most common sleep complaint in America, affecting up to 40 percent of adults. A recent nationwide survey found that one in five Americans takes a prescription or OTC sleep aid at least once a week—and 63 percent of them experience side effects.

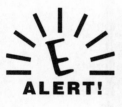

Insomnia can be triggered by several medications, including cold and allergy meds (antihistamines and decongestants), hypertension and heart disease drugs, birth control pills, thyroid medicines, and asthma medications. Caffeine is an obvious cause for insomnia, but it's found in many places beyond your coffee cup, including some OTC pain relievers.

Herbalism has some gentler remedies to offer:

- **Chamomile** (*Matricaria recutita*)

  Chamomile flowers have been used to make bedtime teas for centuries; they contain mildly sedating compounds, as well as chemicals that reduce anxiety.

- **Kava** (*Piper methysticum*)

  Research shows that this herb can be as effective as the drug Valium in creating the changes in brain waves that help you fall—and stay—asleep.

- **Lavender**
  (*Lavandula angustifolia*)

  Lavender oil is used topically as a sedative and antianxiety agent. Research shows it can promote relaxation and induce sleep in people of all ages. In one study, people who used lavender in aromatherapy (they inhaled it or applied it to their skin) before going to bed reported feeling more refreshed in the morning.

- **Lemon balm**
  (*Melissa officinalis*)

  Lemon balm is a mild sedative and stress reliever. Research shows it can quell anxiety and promote sleep.

- **Passionflower**
  (*Passiflora incarnata*)

  Passionflower is a mild sedative and sleep aid.

- **Valerian**
  (*Valeriana officinalis*)

  Valerian is a mild sedative and tranquilizer. Studies show that its chemical compounds can have a direct affect on gamma-aminobutyric acid (GABA), a brain chemical that controls arousal and sleep. Taking valerian can shorten the time it takes you to fall asleep (sleep latency) and improve your sleep quality.

Soothing Skin Inflammation

Inflammatory skin problems often develop when the skin's production of sebum (oil) or skin cells—or both—has gotten out of control. There isn't any clear cause for these problems, although many seem to involve an allergic or abnormal immune response. But we do know that there are plenty of contributing factors, including stress, infection, and certain pharmaceuticals.

Three of the most common skin inflammations are rosacea, eczema, and psoriasis. Conventional medicine treats eczema and psoriasis with a slew of medications. They include oral antihistamines like OTC diphenhydramine (Benadryl) and prescription-only hydroxyzine (Vistaril), plus topical steroids like OTC hydrocortisone (Cortaid) and prescription triamcinolone (Kenalog) and betamethasone (Betatrex). Topical immunomodulating drugs like prescription-only tacrolimus (Protopic) and pimecrolimus (Elidel) are sometimes used for resistant cases of eczema.

Oral antihistamines often cause sedation. Topical and oral steroids can cause thinning of the skin and increased risk of infections. Tacrolimus and pimecrolimus have been associated with increased risk of cancer and immune system suppression. Herbal treatments, which can be used in conjunction with conventional treatments, include these:

- **Aloe**
  (*Aloe vera*)

  Aloe vera is the herb of choice for inflammatory skin conditions and has proven antibacterial and antioxidant effects. In one study, aloe cream cleared psoriasis outbreaks in nearly everyone who used it.

- **Chamomile**
  (*Matricaria recutita*)

  Research shows that topical applications can relieve the inflammation and itching of chronic dermatitis as well as hydrocortisone creams— and better than nonsteroidal drugs.

- **Gotu kola**
  (*Centella asiatica*)

  Gotu kola is well known in Ayurvedic and Chinese medicine for its skin-repairing abilities. Research suggests that topical extracts can relieve symptoms of psoriasis.

- **Licorice**
  (*Glycyrrhiza glabra*)

  Licorice has soothing emollient and wound-healing effects and can help relieve the symptoms of inflammatory skin problems like dermatitis and rosacea. Studies on dermatitis patients show that topical licorice extracts relieve the itching, inflammation, and discomfort better than hydrocortisone.

- **Saint John's wort**
  (*Hypericum perforatum*)

  Saint John's wort is a powerful weapon against many skin disorders, and studies show that topical applications reduce the severity of several inflammatory skin diseases.

Oral Care

Your mouth is more than a passageway for food, oxygen, and words: It's also home to your teeth, gums, and other tissues, all necessary for normal eating, breathing, speaking, and smiling. Things that can go wrong in your mouth include tooth decay and cavities, gum disease, sores on the gums or other soft tissues (mucosa), and bad breath (halitosis).

Conventional dentistry recommends you fight cavities, gum disease, and halitosis with regular flossing and brushing with a toothpaste that contains fluoride, which is a mineral that prevents cavities by bonding to the tooth surface and attracting other minerals (a process called remineralization) and inhibiting the ability of bacteria to create acid.

Standard treatments for canker sores involve topical anesthetics like lidocaine or benzocaine or mouthwashes made with the antiallergy drug diphenhydramine, all of which can cause irritation. Halitosis sufferers sometimes use mouthwashes and rinses made with antiseptics like hydrogen peroxide, cetylpyridinium chloride, or alcohol, which kill bacteria but can also damage tissue and create even fouler breath; cetylpyridinium chloride and diphenhydramine can also stain the teeth.

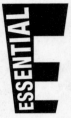

Chewing on a sprig of fresh peppermint (*Mentha x piperita*), spearmint (*Mentha spicata*), or most any mint can clean your teeth and freshen your breath quicker than anything that comes in a tin—and doesn't fill your mouth with sugar, which can make bad breath even worse. Chewing on parsley (*Petroselinum crispum*) has the same effect, minus the minty flavor.

Here are some herbs that can help foster oral health:

- **Calendula** (*Calendula officinalis*)
  Calendula is an antibacterial and anti-inflammatory that's been proven to soothe and heal inflamed mucosa in your mouth.

- **Clove** (*Syzygium aromaticum*)
  Clove oil is a potent antibacterial, and research shows it's comparable to the pharmaceutical anesthetic benzocaine, which makes it an effective remedy for canker and sores. (Diluted, it also works as a germ-killing mouthwash.)

- **Goldenseal** (*Hydrastis canadensis*)
  Goldenseal is a proven antibacterial that makes an effective mouthwash for preventing canker sores and halitosis.

- **Neem** (*Azadirachta indica*)
  In Ayurvedic medicine, neem is used as a toothpaste and mouthwash. Modern research confirms this practice, showing that neem effectively kills bacteria and reduces plaque.

- **Peppermint** (*Mentha x piperita*)
  Peppermint works as an antibacterial and antiseptic (and it tastes really good). It's used in mouthwashes and other oral care products.

- **Tea** (*Camellia sinensis*)
  Tea contains polyphenols, which kill bacteria (and inhibit their ability to form plaque) and also seem to make the teeth more resistant to the acid that causes decay.

- **Isatis** (*Isatis tinctoria*)
  Taken in combination with astragalus (*Astragalus membranaceus*), isatis accelerates the healing of canker sores.

CHAPTER 14

Emergencies
and First Aid

Accidents will happen—and probably when you least expect them. Accidents and unintentional injuries send more than 30 million Americans to the doctor's office each year and close to the same number to the emergency room. Lots of mishaps occur at home (cuts and burns are common household injuries) and in the great outdoors (think insect bites and stings, ankle twists, and sunburns). Luckily, herbs offer lots of emergency aid, helping to relieve pain and other unpleasant symptoms and speed recovery.

Hurry! Do Something!

Unlike chronic illnesses, accidents and injuries are sudden, often unexpected, and require immediate action. First aid is just what its name implies: the immediate assistance given to an injured or sick person. Perhaps the most important part of first aid is being prepared—having the tools and skills you need to assess the situation, determine the best course of action (treat the problem yourself or call for help), and then follow it.

Conventional medicine recommends that you keep some basics on hand, including these:

- Antiseptic solution, like hydrogen peroxide, providone-iodine (Betadine), or benzalkonium chloride (Bactine), to clean wounds and kill germs
- Antibiotic ointment, such as bacitracin/neomycin/polymyxin B (Neosporin), to prevent infection in cuts and other superficial skin injuries
- Antidiarrheal medication, such as loperamide (Imodium) or bismuth subsalicylate (Kaopectate, Pepto-Bismol)
- Over-the-counter (OTC) oral antihistamine like loratadine (Claritin) and diphenhydramine (Benadryl), to stop itching
- OTC oral pain reliever (analgesic), such as acetaminophen (Tylenol), or nonsteroidal anti-inflammatory drugs (NSAIDS) like aspirin and ibuprofen (Advil)
- OTC topical anesthetic, like lidocaine (Topicaine) or benzocaine (Solarcaine, Americaine), to stop pain and/or itching
- OTC topical anti-inflammatory/anti-itch remedy, such as hydrocortisone (Cortaid) or diphenhydramine (Benadryl), to stop itching
- Insect repellant made with N-diethyl-meta-toluamide (DEET) or permethrin, found in Off! and Repel brands, to keep biting insects away

You'll most likely buy the same types of products whether you use conventional or herbal items to stock your first-aid kit. But choosing herb-based instead of chemical-laden supplies can be very helpful—both for you and the person you're assisting.

For example:

- Topical antibiotics can cause skin reactions and (more alarming) contribute to the development of antibiotic-resistant bacteria.
- Topical antiseptics can inhibit wound healing if used long term (large doses of providone-iodine can interfere with thyroid functioning). Benzalkonium chloride can irritate skin, lungs, and mucous membranes.
- Conventional antidiarrheal meds can cause constipation and cramping and may interact with other drugs.
- Oral antihistamines can cause weakness, irregular heartbeat, headaches, and nervousness.
- Acetaminophen can cause liver damage (especially if you regularly drink alcohol or coffee); aspirin and other NSAIDS can cause gastrointestinal bleeding, stomach and intestinal damage, tinnitus (ringing in the ears), and heart problems.
- Topical pain relievers can cause swelling, skin irritation, and irregular heartbeat.
- Topical itch remedies can cause a variety of side effects: Corticosteroids can cause skin reactions and can also impair wound healing and increase your chances of infection; antihistamines can cause redness, swelling, and other skin problems.
- Chemical insect repellants are neurotoxins and have been linked to skin and neurological reactions. Combining DEET with a chemical sunscreen can increase the amount of DEET that's absorbed into your skin, which can be toxic.

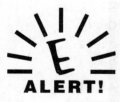

Bismuth subsalicylate is the key ingredient in Pepto-Bismol, one of the bestselling OTC drugs in the United States. It's an effective remedy for nausea, diarrhea, and heartburn, but it can interact dangerously with many other drugs, including prescription blood thinners, pain relievers, and diabetes drugs as well as nonprescription pain and cold medicines.

Herbal Alternatives

In contrast to the pharmaceuticals in an average medicine cabinet, herbal first-aid remedies are generally free of side effects and in many cases perform as well or even better than the commercial drugs.

Compared to the conventional medicines that are based on a single active chemical, herbs contain many constituents. In fact, some experts think that it's this synergy that makes plant medicines superior to drugs made in a lab. Because they have so many compounds acting at once, they're much less likely to cause the side effects you see when you've got a single foreign agent in the body.

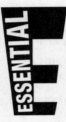

Garlic (*Allium sativum*) is a staple in any herbal first-aid kit. It's a classic remedy for cuts and other abrasions, and modern research has confirmed its antimicrobial and wound-healing properties. Garlic extracts are also good at preventing or minimizing scars—and they're the key ingredient in the OTC scar medicine Mederma—and even work as a bug repellant.

Herbs can also outperform conventional remedies that incorporate more than one active ingredient, such as the first-aid sprays that combine a pain-relieving agent with an infection-fighting chemical, because the herb is almost always kinder to the skin. There are certainly herbs capable of doing harm, but the ones that have been used, time and time again, to treat injuries have been proven to be safe and effective (and generally side effect-free) remedies.

Most herbs contain hundreds of chemical constituents, or phytochemicals, many of which have therapeutic or medicinal value to humans. In many cases, the various constituents in an herb fit perfectly with the first-aid task at hand. For example, a burn might require pain relief as well as a reduction in inflammation and thus would be well served by an herb with both analgesic and anti-inflammatory properties, like calendula (*Calendula officinalis*) or chamomile (*Matricaria recutita*).

A cut or scrape could also use some antibacterial action, so you might use barberry (*Berberis vulgaris*) or tea tree (*Melaleuca alternifolia*), both of which can effectively relieve pain, reduce inflammation, and kill germs. Or maybe you have an injury that needs a styptic (something to stop bleeding) as well. In that case, you can reach for aloe (*Aloe vera*) or horsetail (*Equisetum arvense*).

Bumps and Bruises

When your body suffers an impact, it can leave a contusion or hematoma (also known as a plain old bruise), which involves localized discoloration, swelling, and inflammation. If you take a fall or bump into something hard enough, the tiny blood vessels just under the skin will rupture, and your skin will develop the telltale black-and-blue color as blood leaks into the surrounding tissues and gets trapped there.

In most cases, bruises are not a big deal and will clear up within a couple weeks. However, if you experience severe pain and swelling, see a health care provider, as this may be a sign of a more serious injury. You also should see a doctor if you sustain a black eye that's accompanied by bleeding within the eye, which can cause serious damage to your cornea (the transparent outer surface of your eye).

Conventional and Herbal Answers

Conventional medicine typically treats bruises, bumps, and other injuries that don't break the skin with OTC meds: oral analgesics and NSAIDs, which can cause gastrointestinal problems, and topical painkillers, which can cause skin irritation and other side effects. Several herbs have been used traditionally, both internally and topically, to treat bruises:

- **Arnica**
  (*Arnica montana*)

  Arnica is the classic European herb for bruises and muscle aches and is used as a conventional herbal treatment (for topical application only) as well as a homeopathic remedy, which is extremely dilute (homeopathic preparations are the only safe way to use arnica internally). Studies show it has anti-inflammatory and anticlotting effects, meaning it can reduce swelling and speed the body's efforts to clear away trapped blood.

- **Comfrey** (*Symphytum officinale*)
- **Turmeric** (*Curcuma longa*)

Comfrey is a time-honored topical treatment for bruises (especially the deeper ones that affect muscle fibers). Modern research shows it can improve the pain and tenderness of contusions and muscle injuries. Turmeric relieves inflammation—and the pain and swelling that goes with it—thanks to its chemical constituent curcumin. It's used externally to treat bruises and other skin and muscle injuries.

Burns and Sunburns

A burn is an injury to the skin that can be caused by several things, including heat, chemicals, radiation (such as sun exposure), and electricity. Most burns are minor—you've accidentally touched a hot stove or spent too much time in the sun—and can be treated at home.

Doctors classify burns according to the amount of damage they've caused. A first-degree burn affects just the top layer of skin (the epidermis) and is by far the most common type. A first-degree burn will be red and painful and will blanch (turn white) when you press on it. It may swell a bit and might peel within a day or two, and will probably heal within a week.

ESSENTIAL

Your risk for sunburn depends on the time of day and year (sunburns are more likely on summer days, between 10 A.M. and 2 P.M.), your latitude and altitude (being closer to the equator and farther from sea level means more radiation), and what you're doing (skiing and swimming are done around water and snow, which reflect burning rays).

Second-degree burns affect more layers of skin. The skin will blister and be red and swollen, and will take a few weeks to heal. (These burns are more prone to infection, so you should probably see your health care provider.) Third-degree burns, the most severe, affect all layers of the skin and possibly other tissues as well, and take months to heal. These burns always require medical attention.

Sunburn is a type of radiation burn caused by UV, or ultraviolet, light. You can get one from a tanning bed or booth as well as from the real thing.

Most often, sunburns are minor (first-degree burns) that make you uncomfortable for a day or so. Occasionally, you can get a second-degree burn from sun exposure, meaning blistering, more pain, and a longer recovery time.

Conventional remedies for minor burns include topical anesthetics/ analgesics and oral pain relievers such as NSAIDs. Burns that might get infected are treated with topical antiseptics and antibiotics, which can inhibit healing and cause skin reactions. Here are some herbal alternatives:

- **Aloe**
  (*Aloe vera*)

  The gel from this cactus-like plant is legendary as a burn remedy. Research shows it improves circulation in superficial blood vessels, inhibits inflammation, and promotes tissue repair.

- **Calendula**
  (*Calendula officinalis*)

  Calendula, a.k.a. the marigold, has both astringent and anti-inflammatory properties and is another classic burn remedy. Studies show it also has antiedemic, analgesic, and wound-healing properties.

- **Lavender**
  (*Lavandula angustifolia*)

  The essential oil of lavender is a gentle anesthetic and anti-inflammatory with real skin-healing powers. Research shows it can relieve swelling and pain in minor burns.

- **Saint John's wort**
  (*Hypericum perforatum*)

  Saint John's wort is used topically to treat burns and other superficial skin injuries. It possesses antimicrobial, antioxidant, and anti-inflammatory constituents, and research shows it can modulate the immune response to burn injury in order to speed healing. (Ironically, taking Saint John's wort orally can increase your susceptibility to sunburn, so be sure to use sunblock.)

- **Witch hazel**
  (*Hamamelis virginiana*)

  Witch hazel is a cooling, soothing remedy for burns (and all types of cuts, scrapes, and other skin injuries). Research shows it can reduce skin inflammation in sunburned people. It also works as a styptic (it stops bleeding).

The Travails of Travel

Hitting the road (or the water or skies) can mean big adventure—and big health issues, too. For some people, just the act of flying or riding in a moving car or boat can bring on nausea. For others, new foods (and new bacteria and other pathogens) can spell disaster. Or it could be the altitude that does them in.

Travelers' Tummies

Some people develop traveler's diarrhea when they venture away from home. The condition generally lasts just a few days—if yours goes on for more than a week (or if you become dehydrated), talk to a doctor. Many cases are caused by microbial infection (also known as food poisoning), which often includes vomiting along with diarrhea.

ESSENTIAL

> When you're traveling, look for dishes prepared with these culinary herbs: oregano (*Origanum vulgare*), rosemary (*Rosmarinus officinalis*), thyme (*Thymus vulgaris*), clove (*Syzygium aromaticum*), and cinnamon (*Cinnamomum verum, C. aromaticum*). Research has shown that they all possess antimicrobial action that can kill many foodborne pathogens.

Vomiting can also be caused by motion sickness (a.k.a. seasickness), which happens when your inner sense of balance gets thrown out of whack. Most cases will resolve themselves, but if you're experiencing other symptoms (such as vomiting blood or severe pain), see a doctor.

Conventional antidiarrheal medications include loperamide (Imodium) and bismuth subsalicylate (Kaopectate, Pepto-Bismol), both sold over the counter. Loperamide can cause constipation and cramping. Bismuth subsalicylate can interact with other drugs (including OTC pain relievers and cold medicines) and can exacerbate ulcers. Motion sickness is treated prophylactically with antihistamines—OTC drugs like meclizine (Bonine) or dimenhydrinate (Dramamine) or prescriptions like scopolamine (Transderm Scop)—which can cause sedation and headaches. Nausea and vomiting are treated with OTC antiemetic (antinausea) drugs like bismuth subsalicylate. Here are some herbal alternatives:

- **American ginseng** (*Panax quinquefolius*) American ginseng is known for its antinausea abilities. Research has shown that it can prevent nausea and vomiting before they start (without the side effects of conventional motion sickness meds).

- **Ginger**
  (*Zingiber officinale*)

  This is a classic herbal remedy for nausea (including motion sickness), diarrhea, and other gastric complaints. In the lab, it's been shown to relieve cramping and kill foodborne *Salmonella* bacteria. Ginger is also available almost anywhere—it's used as both a medicine and a spice throughout the world.

- **Juniper**
  (*Juniperus communis*)

  This traditional Native American digestive remedy contains several chemicals with antidiarrheal and antimicrobial properties.

- **Psyllium**
  (*Plantago ovata,*
  P. psyllium)

  Psyllium, which is best known as a constipation remedy, is also an effective antidiarrheal. In the lab, it's been proven as effective as the drug loperamide, without the side effects.

Altitude Sickness

If you travel to an altitude that's significantly higher than what you're used to, you might develop altitude sickness, a condition that can involve headaches, shortness of breath, weakness, fatigue, and stomach upset. At higher altitudes, lower air pressure and less oxygen can create hypoxia, or a shortage of oxygen reaching your tissues, triggering problems in your brain, blood vessels, and lungs.

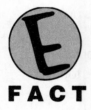

FACT

Different people experience altitude sickness at different elevations, many starting at around 6,000 feet above sea level. In most cases, altitude sickness gets better on its own, as you get acclimated to the elevation (or climb back down again). But extreme cases can result in serious problems, even coma and death.

Conventional doctors sometimes prescribe the drug acetazolamide (Acetazolamide) to prevent and treat altitude sickness, but its side effects include nausea and vomiting. Herbs offer a simpler solution:

- **Asian ginseng**
  (*Panax ginseng*)

  Used for centuries in Chinese medicine as an adaptogen—an herb that can help the body deal with stress—Asian ginseng can lessen the effects of altitude (specifically, the shortage of oxygen and extreme temperatures).

- **Ginkgo**   Ginkgo boosts circulation throughout the body, especially to the brain,
  (Ginkgo biloba)   and can increase tolerance for low-oxygen environments. Research
  shows it can significantly reduce altitude sickness symptoms, including
  headache, fatigue, and respiratory difficulties.
- **Reishi**   This medicinal mushroom is another Asian adaptogen and altitude aid.
  (Ganoderma lucidum)   Research suggests that reishi extracts improve the body's consumption
  and use of oxygen and prevent the damage caused by hypoxia.

Scrapes, Cuts, and Other Abrasions

You can injure your skin anywhere: wielding a knife in the kitchen, shuffling papers in the office, or playing with your kids in the park. You also can develop blisters—fluid-filled pouches of skin created by friction—when hiking on vacation or just wearing a new pair of shoes around your neighborhood. Whenever you break the structural integrity of your body's outermost layer, you're damaging skin (and possibly nerves and muscle fibers) and opening the door to infection.

Minor abrasions can be taken care of with a little soap and water and perhaps a bandage. Wounds that are bleeding (or hurt) a lot might require stronger measures. And if the bleeding doesn't stop after a few minutes or if the would is very big and/or deep, you should see a doctor.

Conventional medicine typically treats minor skin injuries with topical antiseptics like hydrogen peroxide, topical anesthetics like benzocaine, topical antibiotics such as bacitracin/neomycin/polymyxin B, and oral pain relievers like acetaminophen or NSAIDs. Here are some herbal alternatives:

- **Barberry**   Barberry contains the chemical berberine, which has strong antimi-
  (Berberis vulgaris)   crobial and painkilling action. Berberine is also found in goldenseal
  (Hydrastis canadensis).
- **Eucalyptus**   Eucalyptus oil contains antimicrobial, analgesic, anesthetic, and antisep-
  (Eucalyptus globulus)   tic constituents, so it can relieve pain and prevent infection.
- **Gotu kola**   A natural anti-inflammatory and antibacterial, gotu kola is used through-
  (Centella asiatica)   out India and much of Asia to treat wounds and skin infections. Modern
  research shows it stimulates new cell growth and the production of col-
  lagen, the major protein in skin and connective tissue, which speeds
  healing and minimizes scarring.

- **Horsetail**
  (*Equisetum arvense*)

  Horsetail is an analgesic, astringent, antiseptic, and styptic (it stops bleeding) and has been used for centuries by Native Americans to treat superficial skin injuries. In the lab, it's shown antimicrobial action against *Streptococcus* and other types of bacteria and fungi that can infect wounds.

- **Marshmallow**
  (*Althaea officinalis*)

  Marshmallow contains antibacterial and anti-inflammatory constituents. It soothes irritated and damaged skin and forms a protective layer to seal out germs and help the skin repair itself.

- **Yarrow**
  (*Achillea millefolium*)

  Topical applications of yarrow can stop bleeding, reduce inflammation, and prevent infection—like an herbal Band-Aid.

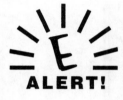

Although you'll find it in practically any first-aid kit in America, hydrogen peroxide is not such a great antimicrobial—and it can actually delay healing of wounds and other skin abrasions. Even very low doses have been linked to neurological, respiratory, and gastrointestinal problems (and high doses have been linked to cancer).

Sprains and Strains

Sprains and strains can strike almost anyone: athletes, weekend warriors, and travelers. A sprain is an injury to the ligaments, which attach muscle to bone; a strain is an injury to a tendon, which attaches a muscle to another muscle, or to the muscle itself.

If you sprain something (the most common site for a sprain is the ankle), you might hear a popping sound, but you'll definitely experience almost immediate swelling and pain. If you've strained a muscle or tendon (what many people call a "pulled muscle"), you'll feel immediate pain, and, over the next few hours, increasing stiffness and possible swelling. Both types of injury occur when the tissue is pulled past its normal range of motion and is either stretched or torn in the process.

Both sprains and strains can be handled at home, unless they are very painful or prevent you from walking or moving the injured area at all. Conventional medicine generally uses OTC pain relievers and anti-inflammatories.

Very painful injuries might be treated with a prescription-strength topical NSAID such as diclofenac (Flector Patch), which can cause skin reactions like itching and burning. Here are some herbal alternatives:

- **Arnica**
  (*Arnica montana*)

  Arnica is a classic remedy for soft-tissue (muscle) injuries. It's used topically (as an ointment or cream) and orally (as a homeopathic remedy) and possesses both anti-inflammatory and analgesic effects. Research shows it can reduce pain and inflammation in patients following surgical reconstruction of knee ligaments.

- **Comfrey**
  (*Symphytum officinale*)

  This herb is used topically to treat injuries to muscles, tendons, and ligaments. Recent research shows that a topical comfrey treatment reduced pain and swelling and restored mobility to sprained ankles better than the prescription NSAID diclofenac.

- **Pineapple**
  (*Ananas comosus*)

  Pineapples contain the enzyme bromelain, which works as an anti-inflammatory. Research shows it can reduce swelling, bruising, pain, and healing time following injury or trauma.

Itching and Scratching

Plenty of things you encounter both at home and away can cause irritation and itching: bites and stings from insects as well as an inadvertent brush against a toxic plant. Other times, itchy skin is the result of an allergic reaction (see Chapter 9). Most often, it's just a case of bad luck: being near the wrong bug (or bush) at the wrong time.

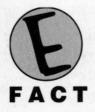

FACT

Several popular culinary herbs and spices contain chemicals with serious bug-repellant powers. Recent studies have shown that extracts of cinnamon (*Cinnamomum verum, C. aromaticum*), clove (*Syzygium aromaticum*), fennel (*Foeniculum vulgare*), and ginger (*Zingiber officinale*) can keep mosquitoes, ticks, and other insects away.

Poison ivy, oak, and sumac contain oils that can cause an itchy, red rash, often involving blisters (you can even have a reaction if you touch something—an article of clothing, even your dog's fur—that's touched the plant, or if you inhale smoke from a fire that contains it).

Several species of bugs—including bees, wasps, and hornets—can sting you, leaving behind venom and sometimes a stinger, plus a welt that's itchy or painful or both. Biting insects, such as ticks, spiders, fleas, and mosquitoes, like to take away something (usually a bit of blood), and leave a bit of saliva that creates a reaction (usually itching and inflammation) in return.

Treatment Options

Conventional medicine typically treats these problems with OTC anesthetics and anti-inflammatory/anti-itch medicines such as corticosteroids and antihistamines. Herbal alternatives include these:

- **Echinacea** (*Echinacea purpurea*)

  Used topically, echinacea is a mild anesthetic and antiseptic that fights infection and speeds healing. In the lab, it's been shown to reduce inflammation and swelling better than a topical NSAID.

- **Eucalyptus** (*Eucalyptus globulus*)

  Eucalyptus oil works as a topical antiseptic and painkiller; it can relieve pain and itching, speed healing, and prevent infection.

- **Sangre de Grado** (*Croton lechleri*)

  This South American tree is known for its anti-inflammatory and wound-healing prowess. Research shows it can relieve the pain and itching caused by all sorts of insects—including fire ants, wasps, and bees—and poisonous plants. It's also good for treating cuts and scrapes.

- **Witch hazel** (*Hamamelis virginiana*)

  A powerful astringent, witch hazel can dry up "weeping" rashes and create a virtual bandage over the area by sealing cell membranes and reducing the permeability of surrounding blood vessels. Research shows that it performs better than hydrogen peroxide in helping skin heal (it's also a strong antimicrobial and antioxidant).

- **Tea tree** (*Melaleuca alternifolia*)

  Tea tree oil reduces histamine-induced (allergic) inflammation of the skin and can decrease the welt left from insect bites and stings. It also has antibacterial properties to help prevent infection.

Conventional insect repellants use chemicals such as N-diethyl-meta-toluamide, better known as DEET, to keep biting insects at bay. Products that contain the chemical permethrin, which is both a repellant and an insecticide, can be applied to your clothing and personal items.

DEET and permethrin can be toxic to people as well as insects, and research shows that they might cause neurological problems and most definitely cause skin reactions (permethrin is designed to be used on clothing only—not skin—and many experts advise saving the DEET for your clothes, too). Herbal alternatives include these:

- **Camphor**
  (*Cinnamomum camphora*)

  Camphor (the herb) contains camphor (the chemical), which is a natural insect repellant. It's also an effective pain and itch reliever (approved by the FDA), so you can also use it to treat bites you've already got.

- **Lemon eucalyptus**
  (*Eucalyptus citriodora, Corymbia citriodora*)

  The oil from this Australian native is registered with the Food and Drug Administration and was recently approved as an insect repellant by the Centers for Disease Control.

- **Neem**
  (*Azadirachta indica*)

  Topical neem preparations have been shown to repel several different species of mosquitoes.

CHAPTER 15

Self-Care and Beauty

Over the last few millennia, humans have put a lot of effort into looking good. Primitive people used twigs to keep their teeth clean, the ancients used fragrant and naturally frothing plants to clean themselves, and Roman women dabbed on creams made with olive oil, rose water, and saffron to keep their skin glowing. Many of the ingredients used in modern lotions and potions are the same as our forbears used—and many more are synthetic concoctions that may actually do more harm than good.

How Herbs Can Help Your Looks

Modern cosmetics contain a laboratory's worth of synthetic chemicals, virtually all of which are deemed safe—or safe enough—by the government. Unfortunately, that's not much of a guarantee. Many people choose herbal self-care products over comparable conventional products because of concerns over safety.

Regulation of Cosmetics and Self-Care Products

The rules governing the marketing and sale of personal care products are enforced by the Food and Drug Administration (FDA). Current regulations prohibit companies from selling "adulterated or misbranded" products—things that contain (or are packaged in containers that contain) poisonous or dangerous substances, are spoiled or contaminated, or have labels with false or misleading information. (A big exception to this rule is hair dyes, which are made with known carcinogens.)

They also require manufacturers to list a product's ingredients and any other information necessary for a consumer to make an informed purchase. If a product contains ingredients that are restricted (such as cancer-causing hair dyes or foaming bath agents, which are known irritants), its label must include the appropriate warning.

What the FDA doesn't control is a product's actual composition: what's in it, how (and if) it works, and if it's safe. Unlike drugs and medical devices, cosmetics fall outside the agency's premarket approval authority, meaning the FDA can step in and try to stop the sale of a product or take action against the company that's selling it only after it's been shown to be in violation of the law. Cosmetics firms, believe it or not, are on the honor system when it comes to manufacturing and selling products that are safe.

Why Herbs Are the Better Choice

Of course, herbs and herbal products fall under the same rules (or lack thereof) that the lab-created cosmetics do, and a skin cream made with jojoba (a natural moisturizer) isn't inherently safer than one made with triethylhexanoin (a synthetic). Unless you grow your own botanicals—and control the seeds you plant, the water you give them, and the dirt you plant them in—you can't be completely sure of what you're getting.

As is the case with conventional products, you also can't always trust the label: There's no official definition of "natural" when it comes to consumer goods, meaning a manufacturer can slap a green label onto a products that's entirely lab created. If you're buying packaged products, be sure to read the label carefully. (For more, see Chapter 17).

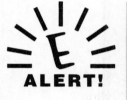

The Environmental Working Group reports that nearly 90 percent of the ingredients in personal care products have not been assessed for safety. Many products contain ingredients that are known toxins and are linked to serious health problems, including cancer and neurological damage. More than 400 products being sold today have been found to be unsafe even when used as directed.

Despite these issues, in most cases, you're still better off with herbs than synthetics. Because they're made with ingredients that are almost always gentler and less likely to cause a reaction than their synthetic counterparts, herbal cosmetics and personal care products generally are a better option.

Healthy Hair 101

Hair grows all over your body, with a few exceptions (including your lips, palms, and soles of your feet), and the average person has about 5 million hairs, most of which grow for between two and six years before falling out and being replaced. Hair—especially the hair on your head—can be a good indicator of your overall health.

Although there are huge variations in what's normal and healthy when it comes to hair (some people have hair that's thicker, curlier, or longer than others), a healthy head of hair is generally shiny, lively, and full. The living parts of the hair—the root, the follicle that contains it, and the sebaceous (oil) gland that's attached to it—are beneath the surface of the skin. The part that's visible, the shaft, which is covered by a cuticle, is dead. Hair gets its color from melanin—the more melanin, the darker the hair. Loss of melanin results in gray or white hair.

Healthy hair requires a few things to stay that way: a good diet with plenty of protein and fat (essential for hair, skin, and other tissues), sufficient sebum, or oil that's produced in the scalp (enough to coat and protect the hair shaft, but not so much that it builds up or collects excess dirt), and a healthy balance of hormones. The good news is that many herbs—whether incorporated in commercial products or used *au naturel*—can keep your hair healthy without all the synthetic ingredients.

Basic—and Better—Hair Care

Many herbs can deliver the same effects—cleaning, conditioning, styling, and coloring—that their lab-created counterparts do, without the hazards.

ESSENTIAL

You can use a simple herbal infusion—a type of "tea" that's not really made of tea (*Camellia sinensis*) but is made the same way—to give your hair color a boost without all the toxins. Try chamomile (*Matricaria recutita*) if your hair is light and amla (*Emblica officinalis, Phyllanthus emblica*) or walnut (*Juglans regia*) if it's dark brown or black.

Everyday Wash and Wear

For centuries, people have used herbs to clean their hair and scalp. Here are a few you can use today:

- **Olive**
  (*Olea europaea*)

  Olive oil is the most common source for castile soap, a vegetable-based cleanser that's gentle for both hair and skin. Castile soap can also be made with other plant oils, including almond (*Prunus dulcis*), jojoba (*Simmondsia chinensis*), hemp (*Cannabis sativa*), and coconut (*Cocos nucifera*).

- **Ritha**
  (*Sapindus mukorossi*)

  The dried fruits of this Asian tree, also known as reetha, soapnut, or Chinese soapberry, also produce a gentle lather. You can find it in some commercial shampoos (imports from India) or mix the powder with water and use it straight.

- **Shikakai**
  (*Acacia concinna*)

  This Indian shrub, also known as soap pod, contains natural saponins, or soap-like chemicals. It's been used for centuries throughout India and Southeast Asia as a gentle shampoo, and it is sold today as a powder (which you mix with water to make a paste) or incorporated into ready-to-use shampoos or oil-based treatments.

- **Yucca**
  (*Yucca glauca*)

  The roots of this Native American plant, also known as soapweed, can be crushed and used as a shampoo. Yucca was also used by the Indians of the Great Plains and Southwest to promote healthy hair growth.

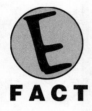

FACT

Many companies are now selling dry shampoos, powdered formulations that can be sprayed into your hair to absorb excess oil and buy you another day without washing. Corn (*Zea mays*)—or, more specifically, cornstarch, which is extracted from corn flour—makes an effective natural alternative. Just sprinkle a bit onto your scalp, then brush it away.

Damage Repair

Hair can be damaged by physical trauma (rough handling or blow-drying), chemicals (coloring or straightening), and environmental factors like UV light. The following herbs can help:

- **Avocado**
  (*Persea americana*)

  Both the pulp and the pit (actually, the oil from the avocado seed) can be used to condition and repair hair.

- **Jojoba**
  (*Simmondsia chinensis*)

  Jojoba oil is considered to be one of the closest herbal cousins of human sebum. It's a classic hair conditioner, used alone or incorporated into commercial products.

Coloring and Styling

Some people like to take their hair beyond the basic (clean and healthy) without venturing into the world of synthetic dyes and styling products, which can leave hair and scalp damaged.

Commercial hair colors are a virtual chemical bath and contain some of the harshest ingredients you can find in an over-the-counter (OTC) product. But you've got some more natural options:

- **Amla**
  (*Emblica officinalis, Phyllanthus emblica*)

  Also known as amalaki or Indian gooseberry, the fruits of this tree are a mainstay of Ayurvedic medicine (used to strengthen the hair and scalp, among other things). Powdered amla fruit can be used as a shampoo (it contains a soap-like chemical) and hair color (it creates an ashy brown shade). Amla oil is used as a hair conditioner, as well.

- **Chamomile**
  (*Matricaria recutita*)

  This is classic treatment for temporarily brightening natural or out-of-a-box blonde hair (it also works on streaks and highlights).

- **Henna**
  (*Lawsonia inermis, L. alba*)

  The best-known natural hair color and one of the earliest cosmetics (Cleopatra was reportedly a fan), henna contains a reddish pigment called lawsone. Henna has been used traditionally around the world to dye hair as well as skin (it's the pigment used in mehndi and other temporary "tattoos").

- **Indigo**
  (*Indigofera tinctoria*)

  Like henna, indigo has a long history of use as a hair and body dye. Once (mistakenly) known as "black henna," indigo actually contains a bluish black pigment—the same one that gives blue jeans their color—that creates a very dark hair color. Some people mix indigo with henna to get a deep brown color.

- **Tea**
  (*Camellia sinensis*)

  Black tea contains mildly astringent tannins (which leave hair shiny) plus dark pigments that intensify and revive black and dark brown locks. The leaves and husks of the walnut (*Juglans regia*) and the leaves of the eclipta, or false daisy, plant (*Eclipta alba, E. prostrata*) are also used to make a rinse for dark brown hair.

ALERT!

Natural henna produces a reddish brown color—there's no such thing as "neutral" or "black" henna—so products promising to deliver other colors must contain additional ingredients. Some manufacturers add chemical dyes or metal salts, which can react with the chemicals in conventional hair products and leave you with green, purple, or otherwise horrific hair. Read labels carefully.

Several herbs work as natural styling products:

- **Aloe**
  (*Aloe vera*)

  Aloe gel is an effective moisturizer for hair as well as skin, and, because it creates a semi-stiff surface when dry, can replace commercial styling gel or hairspray.

- **Avocado**
  (*Persea americana*)

  The rich emollients in avocado pulp work as well as a commercial pomade or sculpting wax, delivering a dose of conditioning at the same time.

- **Marshmallow**
  (*Althaea officinalis*)

  Marshmallow contains humectants (chemicals that attract and hold moisture), which make it a natural hair-styling agent.

- **Nettle**
  (*Urtica dioica*)

  Nettle contains astringent chemicals that are natural body-builders, making it a good stand-in for commercial volumizing products.

- **Psyllium**
  (*Plantago ovata,*
  P. psyllium)

  Psyllium seeds contain mucilage, a slimy substance that does what many commercial gels and mousses do: coats your hair when it's wet and holds it in place as it dries.

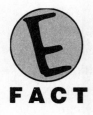

FACT

The average American uses between fifteen and twenty-five personal-care products every day (including several hair care and styling products). But each product you pile on adds more chemicals to your hair and scalp, increasing the chance of a bad reaction (or just a lot of product buildup). In contrast, most herbs work alone or in combination with just a few other ingredients.

Dealing with Dandruff

Dandruff is a broad term for a flaky, sometimes itchy, scalp. In many cases, it's caused by a buildup of hair care products or dry skin on and around the scalp, something that's easily remedied with a change in shampoo and conditioner. In other cases, the flakes are what's technically known as seborrheic dermatitis.

Seborrheic dermatitis is a type of flaking and scaling of the scalp that's caused, ironically, by excessive oil. (The word *seborrhea* means "too much oil.") Seborrheic dermatitis can also create scaly patches on other areas, such as the inside of the ear, face, or torso. A case that develops in an infant is referred to as *cradle cap* (see Chapter 6).

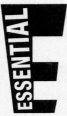

Tea (*Camellia sinensis*) contains astringent tannins along with the anti-dandruff phytochemicals salicylic acid, sulfur, and zinc—close relatives of the chemicals used in commercial dandruff remedies. Steeping a handful of leaves (or a few tea bags) to make an extra-strong infusion gives you an easy, effective after-shampoo treatment for hair and scalp.

Seborrhea symptoms can also be associated with yeast overgrowth, although most experts say the condition itself isn't caused by fungus.

Conventional dandruff treatments focus on removing flakes and fighting inflammation; some are also antifungals. Most of the time, doctors recommend OTC remedies, but severe cases might be treated with prescription-strength shampoos or topical cortisone treatments.

OTC dandruff treatments include shampoos made with salicylic acid (see "Acne and Oily Skin," below), coal tar (a thick, black byproduct of the manufacture of gas and coal that contains known carcinogens), pyrithione zinc, and selenium sulfide; you'll also see antifungal shampoos made with ketoconazole in the dandruff aisle. All can reduce symptoms, but they can cause side effects like stinging or burning and hair loss. Some people also use OTC lotions made with these ingredients, or OTC or prescription steroid creams or lotions, which can cause skin reactions and impair immune function. Here are a few antidandruff herbs:

- **Peppermint**
  (*Mentha x piperita*)

  Peppermint contains menthol, selenium, and zinc—all proven anti-flake ingredients that are also used in conventional dandruff shampoos. Juniper (*Juniperus communis*) contains the same chemicals, along with several antifungal agents.

- **Licorice**
  (*Glycyrrhiza glabra*)

  Licorice contains salicylic acid—the same ingredient in many pharmaceutical dandruff treatments—without all the unnecessary extras. You'll also find a healthy dose of salicylic acid in calendula (*Calendula officinalis*).

- **Tea tree**
  (*Melaleuca alternifolia*)

  Tea tree oil is a potent antifungal that's also drying—perfect to combat seborrheic dermatitis. Research confirms its effectiveness as an effective dandruff remedy.

Too Oily? Too Dry?

Your scalp is covered with hair follicles—about 100,000 of them—most attached to a sebaceous gland, which pumps out sebum. When sebum supplies are right, your hair and scalp are protected from environmental assaults, and they look (and feel) healthy. But if your sebaceous glands are putting out too much (or not enough) sebum, your hair and scalp will look oily (or dried out).

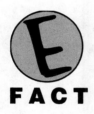

Biotin, a water-soluble B vitamin, is essential for healthy hair and scalp, and a deficiency can cause hair loss, dandruff, and a host of other problems. Biotin supplements can help, but so can eating plenty of biotin-rich plants, like whole grains, legumes, cruciferous vegetables, and herbs like soy (*Glycine max*) and garlic (*Allium sativum*).

Many people have dry skin—on their bodies and faces as well as their scalps—and can experience itching and flakiness (and dry, dull hair) as a result. To restore moisture to parched skin and hair, you can look to commercial products, which most certainly contain ingredients you don't need along with the emollients you do. Or you can try these herbs:

- **Almond**
  (*Prunus dulcis*)

  The oil from this ubiquitous nut—it's grown all over the world—can moisturize both skin and hair without leaving too much grease behind; unlike many other plant and synthetic oils, it's got a light texture and is absorbed into the tissues quickly. Almond oil is also rich in scalp-friendly omega-3 essential fatty acids (EFAs).

- **Cocoa**
  (*Theobroma cacao*)

  Cocoa butter, the semi-solid fat derived from cocoa beans, is a rich emollient and protectant that's great for dry skin. It also contains lactic acid, a proven remedy for rough, scaly skin.

- Flax
  (*Linum usitatissimum*)

Whether used topically or internally, the oil from flaxseeds locks moisture into the scalp and hair and delivers omega-3 acids, which restore the skin's natural moisture balance. When taken orally, omega-3s seem to work best when combined with omega-6 acids, which are found in borage (*Borago officinalis*) and evening primrose (*Oenothera biennis*) oils.

Trying to remedy a case of the greasies generally means hitting the shampoo aisle in search of the strongest shampoo you can find. But that strategy can leave you with dried up, damaged hair and scalp. Herbs offer a better solution:

- Horsetail
  (*Equisetum arvense*)

Horsetail is an astringent herb that was used by several Native American tribes as an oil-inhibiting hair wash. Willow (*Salix alba*) and juniper (*Juniperus communis*) are two more remedies for oily scalp.

- Nettle
  (*Urtica dioica*)

Nettle leaves are also a good source of astringent chemicals, and a nettle infusion makes an effective rinse for oily hair and scalp. Witch hazel (*Hamamelis virginiana*) can produce similar results.

Halting Hair Loss

If you've noticed your hair getting thinner—or showing up in greater-than-normal quantities in your brush or shower drain—you're probably not happy about it. Hair loss, or *alopecia*, can affect anyone, at any age, and can be caused by many things. Some cases will resolve on their own, while others will continue until a large amount of hair (if not every last strand) is gone.

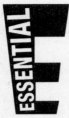

Essential oils—highly concentrated herbal extracts—have been used for centuries to keep hair and skin healthy. Research shows that applying a combination of rosemary (*Rosmarinus officinalis*), lavender (*Lavandula angustifolia*), Atlantic cedar (*Cedrus atlantica*), and thyme (*Thymus vulgaris*) essential oils can significantly improve symptoms of alopecia areata, a type of hair loss that affects both women and men.

At any given time, about 90 percent of the hair follicles on your head are in the growing stage and the others are resting. When its resting phase is over, the follicle sheds its hair and starts growing a new one.

Most people lose between 50 and 100 hairs a day. Losing significantly more than that can mean a few things, including:

- **Hereditary (androgenic) alopecia:** This condition, known as male-pattern and female-diffuse balding, is the most common type of hair loss. Androgenic alopecia is progressive, meaning it won't resolve itself and will only get worse as time goes by.
- **Alopecia areata:** Alopecia areata typically produces round, completely smooth patches on the scalp (and occasionally progresses to complete baldness). Many experts think it's an autoimmune disorder. In most cases, hair returns on its own.
- **Telogen effluvium:** This is a temporary condition in which an abnormally large number of hair follicles enter the resting stage at once, meaning you're losing more than you're replacing. It can be caused by physical or emotional stress, thyroid abnormalities, nutritional shortfalls, and certain medications (including pain meds, anticoagulants, and antidepressants).

Conventional medicine typically treats hair loss with drugs: minoxidil (Rogaine), which started as a prescription but is now available OTC, and finasteride (Propecia, Proscar), a prescription. Side effects of minoxidil can include dizziness or fainting and fast or irregular heartbeat. Propecia can cause sexual side effects. Alopecia areata is often treated with cortisone injections, which can cause suppressed immunity and other problems. But herbal medicine has some alternatives:

• **Eclipta** (*Eclipta alba, E. prostrata*)	Eclipta, also known as false daisy, is an Ayurvedic staple with a long tradition of use as a hair treatment. In modern studies, it's been proven more effective than minoxidil (Rogaine) in promoting hair growth.
• **Garlic** (*Allium sativum*)	Both garlic and its cousin onion (*Allium sepa*) contain oleic acid, a natural antialopecia agent. Research shows that topical extracts of either onion or garlic can help stimulate regrowth of hair lost to alopecia areata.

- **Nettle**
(*Urtica dioica*)

  This plant is a classic European and Native American hair tonic (the indigenous people of British Columbia recognized its ability to promote the growth of long, silky hair). Nettle's astringent properties also make it useful for combating excess sebum, which has been shown to contribute to hair loss.

- **Saw palmetto**
(*Serenoa repens*)

  Taken orally, saw palmetto extracts seem to inhibit the hormonal process that has been blamed for androgenic alopecia.

- **Soy**
(*Glycine max*)

  Soy can help you keep your hair in a few ways: It's used in many commercial shampoos as a gentle scalp cleanser (it contains natural surfactants and astringents), and it also works internally. Soy contains the chemicals inositol and beta-sitosterol, which have been shown to inhibit hair loss.

- **Tea**
(*Camellia sinensis*)

  Regularly consuming green tea (or applying it to your scalp) can produce significant regrowth. Research shows that the polyphenols in tea can help reduce androgenic alopecia.

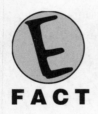

Japanese researchers have isolated chemicals called *procyanidin oligo-mers* from apples (*Malus domestica*) and barley (*Hordeum vulgare*), which they've shown in both laboratory and real-life experiments can increase hair growth by as much as 300 percent.

Acne and Oily Skin

Acne is a disorder of the sebaceous glands that causes clogged pores and pimples on the face (and occasionally the neck, chest, and upper back). Acne occurs when the sebaceous glands produce too much sebum, which can combine with dead skin cells and block the pores. The pores can become infected (most often with bacteria), creating more inflammation.

Conventional medicine treats acne with a three-pronged approach, using medicines that reduce bacteria, unclog pores, and minimize (or remove) oil. OTC remedies include cleansers and treatments made with antibacterial and astringent ingredients like benzoyl peroxide or sulfur and exfoliants like salicylic acid, alpha-hydroxy acids, or retinol. All of these can cause skin irritation and drying. For example, benzoyl peroxide can cause redness and stinging (it's a bleach as well as a bacteria killer).

Prescription treatments include topical retinoids like tretinoin (Retin-A), adapalene (Differin), and tazarotene (Tazorac). Topical antibiotics include erythromycin and clindamycin (Benzaclin, Duac); antibacterials include sulfacetamide (Klaron) and azelaic acid (Azelex). Oral antibiotics include tetracycline, doxycycline, and minocycline. Oral contraceptives such as drospirenone/ethinyl estradiol (Yaz) are also prescribed in some cases. The drug isotretinoin (Accutane) is sometimes prescribed for very severe or resistant cases.

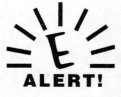
ALERT!

Many chemicals used in acne treatments, including benzoyl peroxide and sodium lauryl sulfate, a cleaning agent, are known irritants that have been deemed "safe" by the FDA because they're used in relatively low amounts in these products. But in slightly more concentrated applications, these same chemicals are routinely used in lab experiments to induce irritation and burns.

Retinoids can cause irritation and increased sensitivity to the sun. Antibiotics can also increase the likelihood of sunburn along with gastrointestinal upset. Birth control pills can cause digestive problems and headaches and increase your risk for several serious conditions (including heart attack and blood clots). Isotretinoin can cause muscle aches—and severe birth defects when taken by women who are pregnant. Here are some herbal alternatives:

- **Calendula**
  (*Calendula officinalis*)

  Calendula is famous for its skin-soothing properties (it contains anti-inflammatory and immune-stimulating chemicals), but it also contains powerful antibacterial and astringent components. An infusion of calendula can replace commercial toners made with alcohol and other potentially drying ingredients.

- **Guggul**
  (*Commiphora wightii, C. mukul*)

  This Ayurvedic herb contains antibacterial, anti-inflammatory, antiseptic, and immune-stimulating compounds. Modern research shows oral doses can be as effective against severe (nodulocystic) acne as the drug tetracycline.

- **Juniper** (*Juniperus communis*)

  Native Americans made an infusion from the branches of this evergreen shrub to use as an oil-balancing hair and skin wash. It has antibacterial, anti-inflammatory, and astringent properties (plus exfoliating alpha-hydroxy acids), making it an effective acne remedy.

- **Tea tree** (*Melaleuca alternifolia*)

  Research shows that a topical tea tree preparation works as well as benzoyl peroxide in clearing pimples, with far fewer side effects.

- **Vitex** (*Vitex agnus-castus*)

  Vitex, one of the best known "women's herbs" used to balance hormonal fluctuations, can be taken orally to prevent or lessen premenstrual breakouts. Red clover (*Trifolium pratense*) is another proven remedy for PMS-related acne.

Saving Face

Unless they're battling acne or another skin condition, most people don't pay much attention to their skin until it starts to show its age. In your thirties, your skin starts losing firmness and volume—and developing lines, wrinkles, and spots instead. And in most people, those telltale signs show up first—and most prominently—in their faces.

Doctors know that as much as 90 percent of what we once thought of as "normal" signs of aging is actually sun damage, or photoaging. Thus, prevention is key (see Chapter 13).

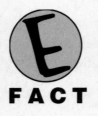

FACT

The fountain of youth might be a coffee pot: Applying extracts of coffeeberries, the unroasted version of the same beans (*Coffea arabica*) that deliver your morning jolt, can significantly reduce wrinkles. Topical or oral doses of plain caffeine also can deliver skin benefits—and research shows that people who regularly drink coffee have lower rates of skin cancer.

Dermatologists talk about ultraviolet (UV) radiation in terms of UVA and UVB rays. UVBs, which are shorter and don't penetrate as far into the skin, are responsible for sunburns and tanning. UVAs, on the other hand, are longer and go deeper into the skin. UVA rays are the biggest culprits in photo-aging and skin cancer.

Both types of UV radiation damage superficial skin cells and destroy the tiny blood vessels that supply nutrients to the skin. Sun exposure generates free radicals, which cause oxidation and play a role in both disease (cancer) and plain old aging.

Conventional medicine offers several pharmaceuticals and treatments to fight the effects of aging in skin. They include antioxidants like prescription tretinoin (Renova) and OTC retinol as well as vitamins C and E, moisturizers like propylene glycol, and exfoliating agents like glycolic acid. These products can improve skin texture and reduce the appearance of lines, but they can also cause skin reactions and increased sun sensitivity.

ESSENTIAL

Many face-saving herbs have been used traditionally in combination remedies and are now being studied scientifically—with great results. For example, a product containing soy (*Glycine max*), grape (*Vitis vinifera*), tomato (*Lycopersicon esculentum*), and chamomile (*Matricaria recutita*) significantly reduced sagging, brown spots, and wrinkles around the eyes, mouths, and foreheads in study participants.

Conventional practitioners also use injectable wrinkle-fillers like hyaluronic acid (Restylane) and collagen and shots of *botulinium* toxin (Botox), which temporarily paralyze facial muscles. Potential side effects include pain and swelling (Botox can cause drooping eyelids or other unwanted paralysis). Herbal medicine offers a few alternatives:

- **Gotu kola** (*Centella asiatica*)
This Ayurvedic herb can strengthen connective tissue and build collagen. Research shows that topical application can improve skin's elasticity and firmness.

- **Grape** (*Vitis vinifera*)
Grape seeds contain high levels of proanthocyanidins, antioxidants up to fifty times more powerful than vitamins E or C. Studies show that grape seed extracts applied to the skin can bond with collagen, boosting skin's elasticity and texture and reducing the signs of aging.

- **Maritime pine**
  (*Pinus pinaster*)

  Taking oral doses of antioxidant-rich pine bark extracts can increase your skin's resistance to sunburn—and counteract the oxidative damage that UV exposure can cause.

- **Pineapple**
  (*Ananas comosus*)

  Pineapples contain alpha-hydroxy acids and other natural fruit acids, which are used topically and have been shown in numerous studies to be an effective weapon against aging. You'll also find them in mango (*Mangifera indica*), papaya (*Carica papaya*), and passion fruit (*Passiflora edulis*).

- **Pomegranate**
  (*Punica granatum*)

  Pomegranate, which is high in antioxidants, can help repair aging skin. Extracts of both the peel and seed (oil) have shown the ability to inhibit age-related collagen loss and speed the production of new supplies.

- **Rose**
  (*Rosa canina, R. spp.*)

  Rose is rich in antioxidants and has one of the highest concentrations of vitamin C in the plant world. Rose oil (from the *Rosa damascena* plant) and rose hips (the fruits left behind after the flower dies) can prevent UV-induced skin damage and act as a natural sunscreen.

- **Tea**
  (*Camellia sinensis*)

  Tea contains piles of dermis-friendly chemicals, including more than sixty antioxidants, at least forty anti-inflammatories, and malic acid (which combines both alpha- and beta-hydroxy acids). Drinking tea and applying it to your skin can protect against sun damage, preventing photoaging and skin cancer.

- **Chamomile**
  (*Matricaria recutita*)

  Essential oil of chamomile has been shown to decrease puffy eyes and dark undereye circles.

CHAPTER 16

Diet, Exercise, and Weight Management

In America, dieting may have replaced baseball as the national pastime. We spend more than $30 billion a year on weight loss supplements (more than a third of dieters have used them). But many people —more than 65 percent of adults at last count— struggle with weight, and most are unaware that plants, including herbs and spices they may already have in the cabinet, can hold the key to healthy eating and weight management.

Weight (and Overweight)

At any moment in America, between 25 and 50 percent of us are on a diet. But we're not making much progress: Our national waistline has been expanding over the past thirty years. Experts predict that 86 percent of adults will be overweight or obese by 2030, a situation that will cost the health care system more than $956 billion. Rates of obesity among adults doubled between 1980 and 2004, and have held steady ever since. Obesity is now recognized as a bona fide disease by experts everywhere, from the American Medical Association to the Internal Revenue Service.

Overweight or Obese?

To put it simply, you're overweight if you weigh more than what's considered healthy for someone of your height, and you're obese if you have too much body fat.

Most doctors agree that having more than 30 percent body fat if you're a woman (or 25 percent of you're a man) means you're obese. Another measurement is your body mass index (BMI), which is calculated using your height and weight: Having a BMI of 18.5 to 24.9 is considered normal, 25.0 to 29.9 is considered overweight, and anything over 30 is obese. To figure out yours, divide your weight in kilograms by your height in meters, squared. Or multiply your weight in pounds by 703, divide that number by your height in inches, then divide again by your height in inches.

In both men and women, obesity has been implicated in a host of health problems, including cardiovascular disease (CVD), osteoarthritis, and several types of cancer, as well as various kinds of disability (obese people are also more likely to die from any cause). For example, experts guess that 20 percent of all cancer deaths in women can be blamed on body weight.

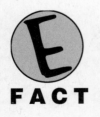

FACT

Proof that less is more: Studies show that consuming 25 percent fewer calories than would otherwise be considered healthy can keep you lean, stave off disease, slow the aging process, and extend your life. Other research shows that eating fewer calories and less fat, especially in the evening, can significantly improve the quality of your sleep.

The numbers on the scale and the BMI table aren't your only concern. Storing fat in your midsection—having an "apple" instead of a "pear" shape—is a known risk factor for CVD and other health problems. In fact, the waist-to-hip ratio measurement is now considered more predictive of chronic health problems than BMI. Measure your waist at the navel and your hips at the widest point, then divide waist by hip measurement. A number that's greater than 1.0 for men and 0.9 for women is considered high risk; 0.9 for men and 0.8 for women is considered average risk.

Obesity is also tied to disorders such as sleep apnea, which is a chronic condition that causes you to stop breathing for short periods of time during the night. Sleep apnea can cause daytime sleepiness and difficulty concentrating—and it's also been linked to heart failure. Sleep apnea is significantly more common in people who are overweight.

ESSENTIAL

Generally speaking, alcohol and dieting don't mix. Booze has no nutritional value but plenty of calories (seven calories per gram of alcohol). But drinking in moderation—one glass of beer or wine a day—can lower your risk of chronic disease, and having your drink with a meal seems to reduce its impact on your waistline.

Nutrition 101

Experts recommend eating a balance of carbohydrates, protein, and fat, with an emphasis on whole foods (vegetables and whole grains) instead of processed ones.

An adult should try to get 45 to 65 percent of the day's total calories from carbohydrates (primarily complex carbs from fruits and veggies, not refined carbs as from sugary or highly processed foods), 20 to 35 percent from fats (mostly unsaturated plant oils instead of saturated animal fats), and 10 to 35 percent from protein. Carbs and protein deliver four calories per gram, and fat has nine calories per gram.

You also should aim for eating 14 grams of dietary fiber for every 1,000 calories you consume. Fiber is essential for healthy digestion and elimination.

You Do the Math

At the most basic level, weight comes down to a simple equation: If the calories you take in through foods and beverages equal the calories your body expends through its essential metabolic processes and the physical activity you do, your weight will remain stable. If the calories in are greater than the calories out, you'll gain weight. If they're less, you'll lose weight.

Calories In, Calories Out

A calorie is a measure of energy. Technically speaking, it's the amount of energy required to raise the temperature of one gram of water by one degree Centigrade. In terms of diet, the calorie is used to show how energy-dense a food is (how much potential energy it contains). The more calories a food contains, the more energy your body can get out of it. Your body breaks down food and gets its energy from it through the process of metabolism.

Your daily caloric needs are based on your gender, age, BMI, and activity levels. The average woman between thirty and fifty years old needs about 1,800 calories a day; a thirty-to-fifty-year-old man needs about 2,200. These are the recommendations for sedentary people—active people and athletes need more.

ALERT!

Scientists know that sweet tastes make us seek more of the same (which creates cravings and late-night ice cream binges). But sugar and other natural sweets (like fruit) can be less problematic than the fake stuff. Recent research shows that people who regularly consume artificially sweetened things like diet soda weigh significantly more than people who eat the real thing.

Unfortunately, most of us consume far more calories than we metabolize. All that extra energy is stored in the body as fat.

A pound of body weight represents 3,500 calories. It doesn't matter where they come from—salads and turkey burgers or French fries and mayonnaise—when you're talking about simple weight gain or loss.

By the same token, it doesn't matter, at least in the short term, if you create your calorie deficit by exercising three hours a day and eating sensibly or by starving yourself and popping diet pills. But in the long run, you'll be able to achieve and maintain a healthy weight only by combining nutritious and balanced meals with regular, vigorous exercise.

GI and TEF

Thanks to the popularity of the Atkins and South Beach Diets, most of us have heard of the glycemic index, or GI. This is a measure of your body's glucose (blood sugar) response to carbohydrate-heavy foods. High-GI carbs, such as sugars and highly processed grains, are digested quickly and create a rapid rise in glucose; low-GI carbs, such as whole grains and beans, are processed more slowly and produce a gradual blood-sugar increase. The more low-GI foods you eat, the lower the glycemic effect (GE) of your meal—and the more satisfied you'll feel.

The glycemic effect is determined by several factors, including the amount of fiber (higher fiber equals lower GE), fat, and protein on your plate. Generally speaking, a higher GE means a higher BMI.

Another consideration is the thermic effect of food, or TEF (*thermogenesis* is the process by which the body generates energy—or "burns off" the calories you consume). Scientists estimate that TEF—the energy it takes for your body to digest the food you eat—represents about 10 percent of your daily calorie expenditure.

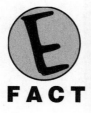

FACT

Adding vinegar to your meal can reduce its glycemic effect—and its effects on your waistline—by as much as 55 percent. Vinegar contains acetic acid, which seems to inhibit your body's response to the carbohydrates you eat, leaving you feeling more satisfied and less likely to eat too much later.

Thus, eating foods with the highest possible TEF means burning more calories without expending any extra effort. Research shows that protein has a TEF that's as much as three times greater that carbohydrates or fat. Protein also produces greater satiety than other nutrients.

Of course, you can't eat all protein—experts recommend getting between 10 and 35 percent of the day's calories from protein. Thus, you've got to make your choices count.

Herbs for Weight Loss

Many herbs have centuries of safe and effective use behind them. Some are being incorporated into over-the-counter (OTC) products, and others can be used as single-herb treatments.

Prescription weight loss medications are reserved for people who have an increased risk of developing health problems because of their weight. That means people with a BMI of 30 or more, or people with a BMI of 27 or higher and an obesity-related condition such as hypertension (high blood pressure) or diabetes (see Chapter 7). These drugs are not supposed to be used for "cosmetic" weight loss, and they're not for people who haven't already tried the old-fashioned diet-and-exercise route.

Herbs, on the other hand, can be used safely and effectively by people with less weight to lose, and most work more gently to achieve the same weight loss effects, with fewer problems. Here are some to try:

- **Konjac** (*Amorphophallus konjac, A. rivieri*)   This Asian tuber, also known as devil's tongue, contains a fibrous compound called glucomannan. Recent trials in obese patients found that it produces a sensation of fullness and aids weight loss (it also lowers cholesterol).

- **Coleus** (*Coleus forskohlii, Plectranthus barbatus*)   This Indian herb, also known as forskolin, appears to stimulate lipolysis, or the breakdown of the fat stored in the body's cells, thus combating obesity.

- **Eucalyptus** (*Eucalyptus globulus*)   Taken internally, eucalyptus leaf extracts appear to interfere with the absorption of fructose, a type of sugar found in many processed foods, thus reducing body fat. (Note that this applies to eucalyptus extracts, not oil, which is toxic when taken internally.)

- **Garcinia**
  (*Garcinia cambogia,*
  G. gummi-gutta)

  Extracts of this pumpkin-shaped fruit contain hydroxycitric acid (HCA), which seems to suppress appetite and inhibit the body's production of lipids and thus help reduce body weight.

- **Gymnema**
  (*Gymnema Sylvestre*)

  This Indian herb is a traditional remedy for overweight. It contains gymnemic acids, which seem to inhibit your ability to taste sweets and delay the absorption of sugar into the blood, therefore keeping glucose levels steady (and cravings low).

- **Maritime pine**
  (*Pinus pinaster*)

  Preliminary research indicates that taking pine bark extracts can inhibit the body's production and storage of fat and may increase lipolysis.

- **Pomegranate**
  (*Punica granatum*)

  Pomegranate leaf extracts contain tannins that appear to lower cholesterol and reduce caloric intake (and body weight).

- **Tea**
  (*Camellia sinensis*)

  Green tea extract has been shown to reduce cholesterol and blood sugar and increase thermogenesis, boosting your metabolic rate.

Building Strength and Endurance

Despite the U.S. epidemic of overweight, many Americans have gotten the memo from the medical community regarding the importance of physical activity and fitness. The government reports that the number of adults who get the recommended amount of physical activity (at least thirty minutes a day, five days a week) and perform the recommended minimum amount of strength training (at least two days a week) has increased in the last few years, especially among women. At the same time, plenty of people are hitting the gym for decidedly different reasons, as both men and women face plenty of societal pressures to be (or at least look) fit—women striving to be thin, men to be strong and muscular.

Store shelves are brimming with supplements promising to deliver ripped muscles, increased strength, and bottomless endurance. Many of these products are targeted at athletes looking to wring just a little bit more out of their training, while others are aimed at sedentary folks looking for a shortcut to a better physique. Substances that improve your exercise performance—they help you run faster, lift more weight, or ride your bicycle longer—are called *ergogenic aids.*

Unfortunately, many of the OTC products being sold in drug and health food stores (and on the Internet) aren't going to do much for you, and some might even be dangerous. For example, experts advise against combining herbal stimulants like guarana (*Paullinia cupana*), bitter orange (*Citrus aurantium*), and caffeine.

However, there are herbs that have been used traditionally and safely, for thousands of years, to improve physical performance and appearance—and that really can help modern folks, too. They include:

- **Asian ginseng** (*Panax ginseng*)

  Research has shown that Asian ginseng can improve exercise performance in cyclists and runners. Other studies show that American ginseng (*Panax quinquefolius*) can decrease muscle damage in athletes.

- **Coffee** (*Coffea arabica*)

  Caffeine has been shown to increase strength, reduce fatigue, and boost performance, particularly in endurance activities and other "submaximal" efforts (less so in sprinting and other activities that use short bursts of energy). It also helps muscles recover, post-workout. Guarana (*Paullinia cupana*), mate (*Ilex paraguarensis*), and tea (*Camellia sinensis*) are also sources of caffeine.

- **Cordyceps** (*Cordyceps sinensis*)

  These inedible and very unappetizing fungi (they grow on insect larvae) are used to treat high cholesterol and fatigue in Traditional Chinese Medicine. Modern studies show that taking cordyceps extracts can increase aerobic fitness.

- **Maritime pine** (*Pinus pinaster*)

  Research shows that taking pine extracts improves exercise performance in treadmill runners.

- **Eleuthero** (*Eleutherococcus senticosis*)

  Eleuthero has demonstrated performance-boosting benefits and seems to allow athletes to train more intensely with less fatigue.

- **Pineapple** (*Ananas comosus*)

  Bromelain, an enzyme extracted from pineapple plants, has been shown to reduce exercise-induced muscle damage and soreness.

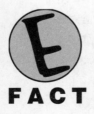

FACT

Men who "bulk up" in order to play better football (or just look beefier at the beach) may be doing long-term harm to their bodies. A new study shows that building excessive muscle mass can contribute to metabolic syndrome, a group of conditions including high cholesterol, elevated blood sugar, and excessive weight gain, which is a proven risk factor for diabetes and cardiovascular disease.

Energy to Burn

America is in the midst of an energy crisis—a physical energy crisis. Scan any magazine (or scroll through the TV channels) and you'd believe that we're all asleep at our desks or just trudging through the day with barely enough energy to make it home, let alone hit the gym or have any brilliant thoughts. The medical term for feeling pooped is *anergia*.

Feeling listless, tired, or fatigued is universal. Everyone has an energy shortfall at some point. Psychological pressures—a stressful job, a jam-packed social calendar—or a shortfall of sleep can leave you stressed out, which drains both your physical and mental energy.

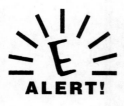

Many people don't realize that fatigue—feeling tired, distracted, or sleepy—can be a sign of dehydration. Being even slightly low on liquids can significantly affect your physical abilities as well as your mental acuity and mood. Be sure you're getting six to eight cups of water a day—more if you're exercising a lot.

In most cases, low energy isn't anything to worry about, but it can be a sign of trouble (such as anemia, depression, or heart or kidney dysfunction). Anergia is not just part of the aging process, nor is it a necessary side effect of modern living. If you feel lethargic more often than not, wake up feeling tired, or nap more than two hours a day, see your doctor.

Commercial "energy" products are often based on stimulants—chemicals that increase your heart rate and other actions of the nervous system to make you feel more alert and energetic.

Many products contain caffeine or synephrine, a stimulant similar to ephedrine (found in ephedra, or *Ephedra sinica*, which was recently banned by the Food and Drug Administration) that comes from bitter orange (*Citrus aurantium*). Stimulants provide a short-lived boost that can leave you feeling worse than before. Too much can cause restlessness and irritability, physical and psychological dependence, sleep disturbances, and other problems.

Some energy bars and drinks also contain lots of protein, which is an essential part of your diet and necessary for optimal functioning (and fighting fatigue). But most people can get enough protein from the foods they eat, and getting more than the recommended amounts won't make you healthier, fitter, stronger, or more energetic. Too much protein can cause weight gain, and way too much can cause kidney and heart problems.

Other energy products contain lots of sugar, which provides a short-term boost but can leave you feeling more tired later.

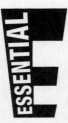

Experts advise keeping your caffeine intake to 300 mg a day from all sources, including supplements. Caffeine is typically listed on a label under the name of its source (often an herb). These include cocoa (*Theobroma cacao*), cola (*Cola acuminata*), grapefruit (*Citrus paradisi*), guarana (*Paullinia cupana*), mate (*Ilex paraguariensis*), and tea (*Camellia sinensis*).

Some energy products also pile on the carbohydrates, which are essential (they're the body's main source of fuel) but plentiful enough in most American's diets. These ingredients won't do much to perk you up either, and also add unnecessary calories. Here are some better ideas:

- **Ashwagandha** (*Withania somnifera*)

  This is a traditional Ayurvedic remedy that's shown the ability to boost energy and offset both physical and psychological stress, including the stress caused by sleep deprivation.

- **Asian ginseng** (*Panax ginseng*)

  One of the bestselling herbs for increasing overall energy, Asian ginseng has been used for centuries to relieve fatigue and offset the effects of stress. Modern research shows it can stabilize blood sugar levels and improve physical and mental performance.

- **Guarana** (*Paullinia cupana*)

  Guarana is a central nervous system (CNS) stimulant and appetite suppressant (it's got about three times the caffeine of coffee). Small doses can boost your energy and endurance and speed weight loss.

- **Maca** (*Lepidium meyenii*)

  Maca grows in the Andes and is a classic remedy for low energy and stress. It's also a CNS stimulant, and research shows it can also keep blood glucose levels steady, increase stamina, and improve both memory and mood.

- **Rhodiola**
  (*Rhodiola rosea*)

Rhodiola can boost physical and mental energy. In separate studies, doctors on the night shift and students at exam time showed better mental performance after taking rhodiola. Other research shows it can increase endurance and reduce physical fatigue.

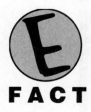

FACT

Savory herbs and spices make a great stand-in for many dietary no-nos, such as salt (you're not supposed to get more than 2,400 mg—about a teaspoon of table salt—a day; most Americans get 3,000 to 7,000 mg). Fragrant spices like nutmeg (*Myristica fragrans*), black pepper (*Piper nigrum*), and turmeric (*Curcuma longa*) can replace salt in some dishes.

Herbs and a Healthy Diet

Food has many connotations: Prestige (filet mignon and expensive cabernet), social consciousness (free-range chicken), moral standards (strictly vegan), or even a busy lifestyle (anything microwaveable). But food should also represent a decision to fuel one's body with the healthiest options around.

ESSENTIAL

Ascorbic acid, or vitamin C, is a powerful weapon against obesity. Separate studies have shown that people who get the recommended levels (that's 75 mg a day for women, 90 mg for men) oxidize 30 percent more fat during moderate exercise than people who don't, meaning skimping on C makes it harder to lose body fat.

Herbs and spices have been used to perk up foods for about as long as people have been eating. Many pack a big nutritional (and medicinal) punch along with their flavorings. They include:

- **Clove**
  (*Syzygium aromaticum*)

  Cloves contain phenols, plant compounds that can regulate blood sugar levels and fight obesity. Cinnamon (*Cinnamomum verum, C. aromaticum*) is also rich in phenols.

- **Garlic**
  (*Allium sativum*)

  Garlic contains sulfur compounds and several other chemicals, including ascorbic acid, chromium, and calcium, that can fight obesity and prevent several obesity-related diseases like hyperlipidemia (high cholesterol) and hypertension.

- **Turmeric**
  (*Curcuma longa*)

  This popular Indian spice contains curcumin, which exerts favorable effects on body composition (read: it reduces body weight and fat stores).

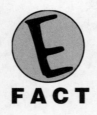

Pyruvic acid, better known as *pyruvate*, is produced in the body through the metabolism of sugars but it is also found in onions (*Allium cepa*), celery (*Apium graveolens*), tomatoes (*Lycopersicon esculentum*), apples (*Malus domestica*), and corn (*Zea mays*). Studies on pyruvate supplements show that it might increase endurance, decrease body weight, and reduce oxidative damage.

Tasty Thermogenics

Several herbs have thermogenic properties—they can increase the body's natural "fat burning" abilities. Here are a few:

- **Cayenne**
  (*Capsicum annuum, C. frutescens*)

  Peppers have been shown to increase the body's ability to burn fat (thermogenesis) thanks to their key constituent, capsaicin. Black pepper (*Piper nigrum*) also has thermogenic properties.

- **Ginger**
  (*Zingiber officinale*)

  Ginger contains several thermogenic compounds, and research shows it can inhibit the intestinal absorption of dietary fat and reduce body weight and blood glucose and lipid levels.

- **Mate**
  (*Ilex paraguariensis*)

  The leaves of this South American shrub are steeped to make a tea, which can promote weight loss by increasing the oxidation of fat and inhibiting the body's ability to store it.

- **Tea**
  (*Camellia sinensis*)

  Green tea contains caffeine and catechins (a type of antioxidant), both of which boost metabolism, increase the oxidation of fat, and help you achieve (or maintain) a healthy weight. Black and oolong teas also contain these weight-loss chemicals.

Fat-Fighting Foods

Many edible plants have proven weight loss benefits—and can easily be incorporated into your diet. They include:

- **Beans**
  (*Phaseolus vulgaris*)

  Common legumes—including black, green, kidney, navy, and string beans as well as soybeans (*Glycine max*) and lentils (*Lens culinaris*)—can slow the rate of carbohydrate and sucrose absorption, significantly lowering the glycemic effect (GE) of your meal.

- **Grapefruit**
  (*Citrus paradisi*)

  This citrus fruit contains fiber and pectin, which create a feeling of fullness, and several chemicals that fight fat. Research also shows that just the scent of grapefruit can reduce your appetite (and food intake).

- **Peanuts**
  (*Arachis hypogaea*)

  Peanuts contain the amino acid arginine, which can lower a meal's GE. Replacing butter with an equal amount of peanut butter or roasted peanuts can reduce your body's glucose response—which affects how full you feel and how much you'll eat later—by as much as 50 percent.

- **Psyllium** (*Plantago ovata, P. psyllium*)

  Psyllium seeds contain lots of fiber and water-absorbing mucilage, which binds to fat and interferes with its absorption.

CHAPTER 17

Safety and Efficacy

Over the past several years, as interest in complementary and alternative medicine (CAM) and herbal medicine in particular has grown, concerns over the safety (and general advisability) of using herbal remedies has been a subject of great concern. The issues of safety and efficacy go hand-in-hand: Who'd want to use something that isn't safe? And why bother about the safety of a remedy that isn't even effective?

Regulation: Who's Minding the (Herb) Store?

Herbal products are classified as either dietary supplements or cosmetics—not medicines—and therefore are handled differently than drugs by the Food and Drug Administration (FDA).

In 1994, Congress passed the Dietary Supplements Health and Education Act (DSHEA), which expanded the definition of "dietary supplement" to include herbs and other botanicals (anything except tobacco) along with vitamins and minerals. The law requires that food products, cosmetics, and supplements be free of "adulteration" and prohibits them from being "misbranded." Manufacturers are also required to use safe ingredients: Anything that was available before 1994 is considered safe, and anything that's been introduced since that time must pass a premarket evaluation by the FDA.

Of course, that's a far cry from the elaborate approval process that would-be drugs face, a fact that leaves some people questioning the inherent safety of herbal products. But herbs don't have it any better (or worse) than any other supplement or cosmetic. The government is surprisingly hands-off in its supervision of the popular (and potentially dangerous) products so many of us pop into our mouths or apply to our bodies every day.

ALERT!

There have been several problems in recent years with imported Chinese patent medicines—standardized, ready-to-use preparations that can be contaminated with pharmaceuticals and other dangerous ingredients. To be safe, ask for remedies that have been manufactured in the United States.

Most Americans assume that the products they buy are being closely monitored—and the mere fact that they're being sold in stores (and not in shady alleyways or on suspicious websites) proves that they're both safe and effective. But both prescription and over-the-counter (OTC) drugs cause more than a million recorded poisonings—and more than 500 fatalities—every year. And cosmetics can cause problems, too. According to the Environmental Working Group, nearly 90 percent of the ingredients in personal care products have not been assessed for safety, and many products contain ingredients that that are known toxins, such as mercury and lead.

Herbal products, in contrast, are almost never involved in cases of serious toxicity or other ill effects. In fact, the vast majority of poisoning cases involving an herbal product involve accidental ingestion by a young child.

The regulations state that herbal products intended to supplement the diet and taken by mouth (such as pills, capsules, or liquids) are classified as dietary supplements. Products that are used externally for self-care or grooming are considered cosmetics.

The FDA can evaluate products and inspect manufacturing facilities at its discretion, but the agency can step in and try to stop the sale of a product (or take action against the company that's selling it) only after the product has been shown to be in violation of the law. Imported herbal products must comply with the same regulatory requirements and are subject to search and sampling by the U.S. Customs Service when they arrive in the country.

What Is—and Isn't—on the Label

Not surprisingly, the government requires very different things from drugs than it does from supplements and cosmetics when it comes to labeling.

Prescription medicines must list the drug's uses, side effects, and other information. OTC drugs are required to provide similar information, including:

- Product name
- Active ingredients (the therapeutic agents)
- Purpose (the product category, such as "antihistamine")
- Uses (the symptoms or condition being treated)
- Directions (how much to take, when to take it, etc.)
- Other information (such as storage guidelines)
- Inactive ingredients (binders, flavorings—the nontherapeutic things)
- Net quantity of contents
- Name and address of manufacturer or distributor

Herbs and other supplements can have significantly less on their labels. The FDA requires the following:

- Product name (plus the words "dietary supplement")
- Nutrition information (a "Supplement Facts" box similar to the "Nutrition Facts" box that's on food packages, which lists the active ingredients, including the part of the plant from which the ingredient is derived)
- Other ingredients (things that are considered inactive or are nonessential nutrients are listed here, below the Supplements Facts)
- Net quantity of contents
- Manufacturer/distributor information (if the product is imported, the label must disclose the country of origin)

In 2007, the FDA issued new standards, termed Good Manufacturing Practices (GMPs), which require herbals and other supplements to be produced in a quality manner, be free of contaminants or impurities, and contain the exact ingredients (in the exact amounts) listed on the label.

This means that you might not be able to tell much from an herbal product's label. For example, a bottle of hawthorn (*Crataegus monogyna, C. oxyacantha*) capsules might include a picture of the herb (a thorny bush covered with white flowers or red berries) but not the condition or body part it's good for (an ailing human heart). Many manufacturers include dosages and guidelines, but not all do.

What Can This Stuff Do?

Dietary supplements are prohibited from claiming to diagnose, cure, mitigate, treat, or prevent a disease—a bit of regulatory red tape that can leave consumers in the dark. But supplement manufacturers are allowed to make these claims on product labels and in advertising and marketing materials:

- **Health claims** mention the relationship between an herb or another ingredient and a lowered risk of a particular disease or condition. For example, products containing vitamins E or C may include a statement on how antioxidants can lower your risk of developing cancer.
- **Nutrient content claims** describe the relative amount of a nutrient or dietary substance in a product. For example, a multivitamin might claim to deliver a full day's supply of a particular vitamin.
- **Structure and function claims** describe how a product may affect the organs or systems of the body but can't mention any specific disease. For example, a calcium supplement's label might say "Calcium builds strong bones," but not "Calcium prevents osteoporosis." Structure and function claims must be accompanied by the disclaimer: "These statements have not been evaluated by the FDA. This product is not intended to diagnose, treat, cure, or prevent any disease."

While some herbs can interfere with certain medications, most can be used without fear of interactions. In comparison, OTC antacids, which are some of the most widely used drugs in the United States, can interact with a long list of other medications, including many those used to treat acne, diabetes, anxiety, thyroid problems, and—ironically—ulcers.

Other Differences

Beyond the regulatory distinctions, herbs and drugs differ in another big way: While drugs contain a specific amount of specific ingredients, plants—even plants of the same species—can vary quite a bit in their contents.

A plant's chemical makeup can be affected by many things, including the environment it was raised in, the way it was harvested and processed, and how it was stored. So while a pharmaceutical company can, at least in theory, control every detail of the pills it produces, herbal products manufacturers must leave a lot to nature.

Research and Scientific Proof

It's been said that herbal medicines and pharmaceuticals arrive at the same destination—the shelf in your neighborhood drug store—from opposite directions. Pharmaceuticals are created in a lab in response to a specific need or to treat a specific condition. Herbs have been around for ages while humans have proceeded, through trial and error, to figure out how to use them.

Preclinical research involves basic science and usually begins with *in vitro* studies, which are conducted on isolated cells (*in vitro* means "within the glass" in Latin). *In vitro* studies gauge a substance's effects on live tissue.

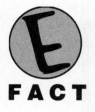

FACT

According to the World Health Organization, ninety-two countries around the world have a system of national regulation for herbal medicines. The United States is one of only a handful of industrialized nations to have no policy. Nearly all countries allow herbals to be sold as OTC drugs, and about half allow herbal medicines to be sold as prescription medicines.

Next, *in vivo* (or "within the living") research uses live animals, often mice and rats, to see what the substance does to a living animal.

Human studies, as you might expect, are experiments conducted on people. They can involve *epidemiological* research, which analyzes data on the use of the herb in a particular group and its relationship to disease and mortality rates, or an analysis of several previously published human trials (called a *meta-analysis*).

Human research also involves *clinical trials*, which compare the substance to a drug or other agent or to a placebo, which is a substance with no pharmaceutical effect (a "sugar pill"), to determine its effectiveness. The best trials are double-blind, meaning that neither the subjects nor the test administrators know who is getting the herb and who is getting the other agent or placebo. This eliminates the risk of prejudice.

Because they must go through a much more elaborate process in order to be approved for sale, pharmaceuticals are much more rigorously tested than herbs (remember, it's much easier to get "dietary supplement" than "drug" status). Thus, the research on many herbs stops at the *in vivo* stage.

However, there have been several important human clinical trials on herbs in recent years, many of which have shown herbs to be safe and effective alternatives to synthetic drugs.

Other Kinds of Evidence

Of course, herbs do have one big advantage over drugs: They've been used safely and successfully for thousands of years. Dose for dose, they are almost always less potent than their pharmaceutical counterparts, meaning they present far less risk of toxicity than drugs do. Many have no known side effects (or very, very mild ones) for people who are otherwise healthy and not taking other medications. Nonetheless, they are medicines and should be treated with care.

ALERT!

Some herbs can interact with cytochrome P450 (CYP), a group of enzymes that are involved in the metabolism of several drugs. There are CYP enzymes that are known to have drug or herb interactions. Be sure to talk with your doctor if you're taking any medications long term, as they might be on the CYP "potential interactions" list.

The Question of Standardization

Some herbs are standardized for a certain level of an active compound, meaning they've been processed in a way that isolates and measures the key constituent or constituents—something that makes it a whole lot easier for consumers to know what they're buying. However, the issue of standardization is fairly controversial.

Medicinal herbs that are sold in Europe are typically standardized to contain a certain amount of the constituent responsible for their therapeutic effect, also known as the *active ingredient* or *marker*. Thus, milk thistle (*Silybum marianum*) is standardized for *silymarin*, the compound that seems to be behind its medicinal effects.

Standardization makes sense for several reasons. From a quality-control standpoint, it allows manufacturers to ensure consistency of their products from batch to batch. It also guarantees that the product contains a therapeutic dose of the medicinal ingredients that made you want to buy it in the first place.

Ideally, the compounds that are used for standardization would be the ones that are responsible for the herb's beneficial effects. In this way, every time you bought an herb in 250 mg capsules, you'd know exactly how many milligrams of the active ingredient you were getting and what effects you could expect.

But in the majority of cases, the exact compounds that are producing the effect is unknown, meaning you can't know which ones to pick for standardization. In many cases, we also don't always know what other compounds, or *cofactors*, must be present in order for the active constituent to do its job.

Consider Saint John's wort (*Hypericum perforatum*), one of the most popular and well-researched herbs around. Scientists continue to debate over which of the plant's many chemical constituents (there are about sixty) is or are responsible for its medicinal effects. A few years back, everyone seemed to agree that it's the *hypericin*, and commercial products standardized for hypericin started appearing. Then researchers began to wonder if another chemical, *hyperforin*, was the real active ingredient. As of this printing, the jury is still out.

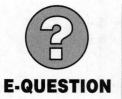

E-QUESTION

How does Saint John's wort work?
We know that Saint John's wort (*Hypericum perforatum*) works against depression, we're just not sure how. Most clinical studies have used preparations standardized for 0.3 percent of a chemical called *hypericin*, but others have used less concentrated products—and others used products standardized for 5 percent of another chemical, *hyperforin*. Studies on both compounds found beneficial results, leaving the question unanswered.

What's more, the practice of standardization itself isn't exactly standardized. Different U.S. manufacturers standardize for different amounts of marker compounds and use different methods of testing.

Meanwhile, many herbalists and natural health practitioners advocate using extracts of the whole herb (or the whole herb part, such as the root) instead of any isolated components. These are called *crude* extracts. Aside from the question of picking the right ingredient to isolate, they argue that this is the best strategy because herbs have been used for centuries as intact organisms, not individual chemicals, and there's evidence that the various constituents in herbs work together synergistically.

Unfortunately, this isn't an ideal solution, either. Because there can be such disparity among crops of plants, there can be enormous variation among their crude extracts—meaning some batches may have higher levels of active constituents than others.

Right now, the best approach seems to be using standardized crude extracts wherever possible. This means you're getting the whole herb and all of its components but are ensured of getting a therapeutic dose of the active ingredient (or at least the ingredient that seems to be the active one). For more on buying herbal preparations, see Chapter 18.

Medical Concerns

If you have specific health issues, including chronic conditions like diabetes or cardiovascular disease, you should use extra care when taking herbal remedies. If you're taking medicines as part of a long-term treatment plan, be sure to get your doctor's approval before using herbs. Some can amplify the effects of medicines and interfere with cytochrome P450 (CYP), an enzyme that's critical to drug metabolism.

Chronic Conditions

While herbs have been used for centuries to help manage chronic diseases and conditions, you shouldn't treat yourself. If you have any of the following health concerns, talk with your doctor before using herbal products:

- Blood clotting problems
- Cancer

- Cardiovascular disease (including heart disease and/or hypertension)
- Clinical depression or another psychiatric condition
- Diabetes
- Enlarged prostate
- Epilepsy
- Eye diseases, such as glaucoma
- Immune system problems
- Liver disease
- Parkinson's disease
- Thyroid disease

Surgery and Anesthesia

If you're scheduled to have surgery, be sure to talk with your doctor about any herbs you're taking. In most cases, she will tell you to stop taking them a few weeks before your operation.

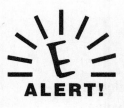

ALERT!

Some herbs can interfere with the results of common lab tests. For example, American ginseng (*Panax quinquefolius*) can conflict with blood glucose tests, and evening primrose (*Oenothera biennis*) can affect your cholesterol levels (and skew the results of a lipid profile). Talk to your doctor about the herbs you're taking before scheduling any tests.

Several herbs, including ginkgo (*Ginkgo biloba*) and turmeric (*Curcuma longa*), can cause problems during surgery by interfering with the anesthesia or increasing the risk of bleeding.

Prescription and OTC Drugs

Many prescription and OTC drugs can interact with herbal products. Herbs can affect the way your body processes a pharmaceutical agent—and vice versa. For example, Saint John's wort (*Hypericum perforatum*) can affect the absorption of certain drugs, increasing the amount that's absorbed in some cases and reducing it in others (meaning you're not getting enough of the drug to treat the condition it's supposed to be treating).

You should talk with your doctor before combining herbs and any pharmaceuticals, but be especially careful if you're taking any of these:

- Antidepressants, antianxiety drugs, or any other psychotropic medications
- Antiseizure drugs
- Anticoagulant/antiplatelet drugs (also known as blood thinners)
- Antihypertensives
- Heart medicines, such as beta blockers or nitrates
- Cancer drugs
- Diabetes medicines

Special Groups

Pregnant women, young children, and seniors all have special concerns—and should take extra care with herbal medicines.

Pregnancy and Breastfeeding

Some herbs are safe for pregnant and breastfeeding women, while others are known to causes problems. Pregnant and breastfeeding women should not take:

- Black cohosh (*Actaea racemosa, Cimicifuga racemosa*)
- Dong quai (*Angelica sinensis*)
- Feverfew (*Tanacetum parthenium*)
- Goldenseal (*Hydrastis canadensis*)
- Juniper (*Juniperus communis*)
- Red clover (*Trifolium pratense*)
- Kava (*Piper methysticum*)
- Sage (*Salvia officinalis, S. lavandulaefolia*)
- Saint John's wort (*Hypericum perforatum*)
- Vitex (*Vitex agnus-castus*)

Pregnant women also should avoid caffeine-containing herbs, such as coffee (*Coffea arabica*), guarana (*Paullinia cupana*), mate (*Ilex paraguariensis*), and tea (*Camellia sinensis*).

Pregnant women can take these herbs, worry free:

- **Ginger** (*Zingiber officinale*)
- **Peppermint** (*Mentha x piperita*)
- **Psyllium** (*Plantago ovata, P. psyllium*)

In addition, aloe (*Aloe vera*), cayenne (*Capsicum annuum, C. frutescens*), gotu kola (*Centella asiatica*), and witch hazel (*Hamamelis virginiana*) can be used topically—and safely—during pregnancy.

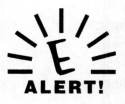

Any medicine, whether it's from a pharmacy or a plant, can be passed from a pregnant woman to her unborn baby or from a nursing mother to her infant. Because there's so little research, some experts advise pregnant and breastfeeding women to avoid taking any herbs orally, with the exception of those specified here.

Babies and Children

Generally speaking, you should stick to herbs with relatively gentle actions when treating children. Don't treat babies or kids with herbs that work as stimulants, stimulant laxatives, strong sedatives, or phytoestrogens. Don't give the following herbs to a baby or young child:

- **Black cohosh** (*Actaea racemosa, Cimicifuga racemosa*)
- **Guarana** (*Paullinia cupana*)
- **Red clover** (*Trifolium pratense*)

Many herbs have a long history of being safe for children. They include:

- **American ginseng** (*Panax quinquefolius*)
- **Echinacea** (*Echinacea purpurea*)
- **Flax** (*Linum usitatissimum*)
- **Ginger** (*Zingiber officinale*)
- **Lemon balm** (*Melissa officinalis*)
- **Licorice** (*Glycyrrhiza glabra*)
- **Passionflower** (*Passiflora incarnata*)
- **Peppermint** (*Mentha x piperita*)
- **Psyllium** (*Plantago ovata, P. psyllium*)
- **Slippery elm** (*Ulmus rubra*)

In addition, the following herbs are safe for children when applied topically:

- Calendula (*Calendula officinalis*)
- Lavender (*Lavandula angustifolia*)
- Rice bran (*Oryza sativa*)
- Garlic (*Allium sativum*)
- Goldenseal (*Hydrastis canadensis*)

Seniors

Many seniors will find that they can use lower doses of many medications—and herbs—as their bodies often process drugs differently than younger people's bodies do. Talk to your doctor to determine the best dosage.

Many of the prescription and OTC drugs used by seniors can interact with herbs. For example, anticoagulant/antiplatelet drugs—also known as blood thinners—can interact with several herbs, including Asian ginseng (*Panax ginseng*), dong quai (*Angelica sinensis*), feverfew (*Tanacetum parthenium*), garlic (*Allium sativum*), and ginkgo (*Ginkgo biloba*).

And the cardiac drug digoxin (Lanoxin, Digitek), also known as digitalis, can interact with several popular herbs, including hawthorn (*Crataegus monogyna, C. oxyacantha*) and Saint John's wort (*Hypericum perforatum*). To be safe, talk with your doctor before using any herbal preparations.

Actions and Interactions

Because they have medicinal properties, herbs should be considered drugs when it comes to interactions. Just as you would do (or should do) when taking prescription or OTC pharmaceuticals, you should make sure that the herbs you're taking aren't interfering with any drugs—or with each other.

Herbs with Sedative Properties

Several herbs act as sedatives (they induce relaxation and sleepiness) and can have an additive effect—that is, they'll increase the action of another agent—when combined with other sedatives, including alcohol.

Don't combine sedating drugs like antihistamines (including those in antimotion-sickness meds) or insomnia remedies with herbs like gotu kola (*Centella asiatica*), kava (*Piper methysticum*), or valerian (*Valeriana officinalis*), which are sedating on their own. Other sedating herbs include:

- **Ashwagandha** (*Withania somnifera*)
- **Calendula** (*Calendula officinalis*)
- **Chamomile** (*Matricaria recutita*)
- **Eleuthero** (*Eleutherococcus senticosus*)
- **Gotu kola** (*Centella asiatica*)
- **Hops** (*Humulus lupulus*)

- **Kava** (*Piper methysticum*)
- **Lemon balm** (*Melissa officinalis*)
- **Passionflower** (*Passiflora incarnata*)
- **Sage** (*Salvia officinalis, S. lavandulaefolia*)
- **Valerian** (*Valeriana officinalis*)

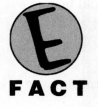

The government requires nonprescription products to carry a "Drug Facts" label that includes the active ingredients, uses, warnings, and directions (dosage instructions). Packaged herbals are simply required to list the product's ingredients on a "Supplement Facts" label (and bulk herbs may have no label at all), meaning you'll have to do your own research before taking them.

Herbal Stimulants

Several herbs contain caffeine or other chemicals that stimulate the central nervous system. They can have additive effects when combined with other stimulants. They include:

- **Asian ginseng** (*Panax ginseng*)
- **Cocoa** (*Theobroma cacao*)
- **Coffee** (*Coffea arabica*)

- **Guarana** (*Paullinia cupana*)
- **Mate** (*Ilex paraguariensis*)
- **Tea** (*Camellia sinensis*)

Herbs and Blood Sugar

Several herbs work to lower glucose levels, but they can reduce blood sugar too much when combined with diabetes drugs, which do the same thing. Herbs with hypoglycemic potential include:

- Alfalfa (*Medicago sativa*)
- Aloe (*Aloe vera*), when used internally
- Asian ginseng (*Panax ginseng*)
- Bilberry (*Vaccinium myrtillus*)
- Cinnamon (*Cinnamomum verum, C. aromaticum*)
- Eleuthero (*Eleutherococcus senticosus*)
- Eucalyptus (*Eucalyptus globulus*)
- Fenugreek (*Trigonella foenum-graecum*)
- Flax (*Linum usitatissimum*)
- Ginger (*Zingiber officinale*)
- Horse chestnut (*Aesculus hippocastanum*)
- Konjac (*Amorphophallus konjac, A. rivieri*)
- Kudzu (*Pueraria lobata*)
- Nettle (*Urtica dioica*)
- Onion (*Allium cepa*)
- Sage (*Salvia officinalis, S. lavandulaefolia*)
- Tinospora (*Tinospora cordifolia*)

Cardioactive Herbs

Several herbs exert a direct effect on heart function, and so should be avoided by anyone with a heart condition (or anyone taking drugs to treat a heart condition). These include:

- Asian ginseng (*Panax ginseng*)
- Coleus (*Coleus forskohlii, Plectranthus barbatus*)
- Danshen (*Salvia miltiorrhiza*)
- Devil's claw (*Harpagphytum procumbens*)
- Hawthorn (*Crataegus monogyna, C. oxyacantha*)

Grapefruit (*Citrus paradisi*) is used as both a medicinal herb and a breakfast drink, but it can cause big problems if it's combined with a variety of medications, including oral contraceptives and prescription allergy, anxiety, and insomnia drugs. Doctors suggest you skip the supplemental grapefruit if you're taking any medications—and wash your medications down with water instead.

Anticoagulant/Antiplatelet Action

Several herbs affect platelet aggregation, or clotting of your blood, and so should be avoided if you're taking medicines that do the same thing, such as clopidogrel (Plavix) and warfarin (Coumadin). You should discontinue using them at least two weeks before any surgery. They include:

- **Andrographis** (*Andrographis paniculata*)
- **Asian ginseng** (*Panax ginseng*)
- **Borage** (*Borago officinalis*)
- **Cayenne** (*Capsicum annuum, C. frutescens*)
- **Chamomile** (*Matricaria recutita*)
- **Coleus** (*Coleus forskohlii, Plectranthus barbatus*)
- **Danshen** (*Salvia miltiorrhiza*)
- **Dong quai** (*Angelica sinensis*)
- **Eleuthero** (*Eleutherococcus senticosus*)
- **Evening primrose** (*Oenothera biennis*)
- **Fenugreek** (*Trigonella foenum-graecum*)
- **Feverfew** (*Tanacetum parthenium*)
- **Flax** (*Linum usitatissimum*)
- **Garlic** (*Allium sativum*)
- **Ginger** (*Zingiber officinale*)
- **Ginkgo** (*Ginkgo biloba*)
- **Horse chestnut** (*Aesculus hippocastanum*)
- **Kudzu** (*Pueraria lobata*)
- **Licorice** (*Glycyrrhiza glabra*)
- **Onion** (*Allium cepa*)
- **Pineapple** (*Ananas comosus*)
- **Red clover** (*Trifolium pratense*)
- **Reishi** (*Ganoderma lucidum*)
- **Turmeric** (*Curcuma longa*)
- **Willow** (*Salix alba*)

ESSENTIAL

Don't combine OTC decongestants with stimulant herbs like mate (*Ilex paraguariensis*) or guarana (*Paullinia cupana*). All of these things can raise your blood pressure and cause other side effects (like increased heart rate, jittery nerves, or irritability).

Hormonal Effects

Some herbs contain chemicals called *phytoestrogens* that act like the human hormone estrogen. Others affect estrogen levels through different mechanisms. Generally speaking, pregnant and nursing women, men, and children should avoid them, as should anyone with a hormone-dependent disease or condition. You also should use caution when combining them with oral contraceptives. They include:

- **Alfalfa** (*Medicago sativa*)
- **Black cohosh** (*Actaea racemosa, Cimicifuga racemosa*)
- **Dong quai** (*Angelica sinensis*)
- **Flax** (*Linum usitatissimum*)
- **Kudzu** (*Pueraria lobata*)
- **Red clover** (*Trifolium pratense*)
- **Saw palmetto** (*Serenoa repens*)
- **Soy** (*Glycine max*)
- **Vitex** (*Vitex agnus-castus*)

Immunity Modulators

Some herbs can affect your immune system, and therefore shouldn't be combined with immunosuppressant drugs. They include:

- Alfalfa (*Medicago sativa*)
- Androgenesis (*Andrographis paniculata*)
- Ashwagandha (*Withania somnifera*)
- Astragalus (*Astragalus membranaceus*)
- Cat's claw (*Uncaria guianensis, U. tomentosa*)
- Cordyceps (*Cordyceps sinensis*)
- Elderberry (*Sambucus nigra*)
- Eleuthero (*Eleutherococcus senticosus*)
- Maritime pine (*Pinus pinaster*)
- Neem (*Azadirachta indica*)
- Reishi (*Ganoderma lucidum*)
- Tinospora (*Tinospora cordifolia*)

Immunity Stimulants

Some herbs increase immune function, and shouldn't be taken by people with autoimmune disorders:

- Barberry (*Berberis vulgaris*)
- Echinacea (*Echinacea purpurea*)
- Goldenseal (*Hydrastis canadensis*)
- Tinospora (*Tinospora cordifolia*)

Herbs and Hyperlipidemia

Several herbs work to lower cholesterol—and can increase the effect of pharmaceuticals that do the same; they also can skew laboratory lipid test results. They include:

- Alfalfa (*Medicago sativa*)
- Flax (*Linum usitatissimum*)
- Garlic (*Allium sativum*)
- Guggul (*Commiphora wightii, C. mukul*)
- Hawthorn (*Crataegus monogyna, C. oxyacantha*)
- Oat (*Avena sativa*)
- Psyllium (*Plantago ovata, P. psyllium*)

Herbs and Hypertension

Several herbs have hypotensive effects and so shouldn't be combined with other blood pressure-lowering agents. They include:

- Andrographis (*Andrographis paniculata*)
- Cat's claw (*Uncaria guianensis, U. tomentosa*)
- Coleus (*Coleus forskohlii, Plectranthus barbatus*)
- Garlic (*Allium sativum*)
- Hawthorn (*Crataegus monogyna, C. oxyacantha*)
- Nettle (*Urtica dioica*)
- Olive (*Olea europaea*)
- Pomegranate (*Punica granatum*)
- Reishi (*Ganoderma lucidum*)
- Valerian (*Valeriana officinalis*)

Others can cause a rise in blood pressure. They include:

- Licorice (*Glycyrrhiza glabra*)
- Sage (*Salvia officinalis, S. lavandulaefolia*)
- Yohimbe (*Pausinystalia yohimbe*)

Liver Concerns

Some herbs can adversely affect liver function—they're potentially hepatotoxic—and shouldn't be used concurrently. They also shouldn't be combined with hepatotoxic pharmaceuticals such as acetaminophen (Tylenol). These agents can also interfere with liver function tests and might exacerbate liver problems in some people. Herbs that can affect liver function include:

- Black cohosh (*Actaea racemosa, Cimicifuga racemosa*)
- Borage (*Borago officinalis*)
- Butterbur (*Petasites hybridus*)
- Cinnamon (*Cinnamomum verum, C. aromaticum*)
- Comfrey (*Symphytum officinale*)
- Gotu kola (*Centella asiatica*)
- Kava (*Piper methysticum*)

The Issues of Allergies

Several medicinal herbs belong to botanical families that, unfortunately, can cause allergies in some people. The *Asteraceae/Compositae* family contains many medicinal plants—and a few common allergens. If you're allergic to ragweed, marigolds, or daisies, avoid these herbs:

- Arnica (*Arnica montana*)
- Artichoke (*Cynara cardunculus, C. scolymus*)
- Butterbur (*Petasites hybridus*)
- Calendula (*Calendula officinalis*)
- Chamomile (*Matricaria recutita*)
- Dandelion (*Taraxucum officinale*)

- Echinacea (*Echinacea purpurea*)
- Eclipta (*Eclipta alba, E. prostrata*)
- Feverfew (*Tanacetum parthenium*)
- Milk thistle (*Silybum marianum*)
- Yarrow (*Achillea millefolium*)

Salicylic acid is part of a group of chemicals called *salicylates*, which occur naturally in many plants and are also produced synthetically for use in a variety of consumer products.

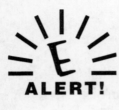

Salicylates are everywhere. They can be found in many skin care products, including acne treatments, perfumes, and sunscreens, as well as aspirin, antidiarrheal medications, toothpastes, and OTC sports creams. They're also in a variety of foods, including berries, red wine, and pine nuts. To someone with sensitivity, even a tiny dose can cause a serious reaction.

Many people are sensitive to salicylates, and so should avoid them in all their incarnations. Skip salicylates if you're taking prescription blood thinners or diabetes medications. Herbs with salicylates include:

- Cayenne (*Capsicum annuum, C. frutescens*)
- Cinnamon (*Cinnamomum verum, C. aromaticum*)
- Clove (*Syzygium aromaticum*)
- Fenugreek (*Trigonella foenum-graecum*)
- Ginger (*Zingiber officinale*)
- Grape (*Vitis vinifera*)

- Grapefruit (*Citrus paradisi*)
- Licorice (*Glycyrrhiza glabra*)
- Peppermint (*Mentha x piperita*)
- Sage (*Salvia officinalis, S. lavandulaefolia*)
- Turmeric (*Curcuma longa*)
- Willow (*Salix alba*)

How to Stay Safe

Here are a few things to keep in mind when using herbs or herbal products:

- **Be informed.** Use resources such as this book and the many organizations listed in the Appendices to research the herbs you'd like to use. Be sure to find out about your individual health needs and not just general guidelines.
- **Talk to your doctor.** Doctors bemoan the fact that very few of their patients talk to them about the herbal products and other supplements they're using. Even if your doctor isn't particularly well versed in herbalism, he should know what you're taking and should be able to advise you accordingly. If you think your doctor isn't open to the use of herbal remedies, find a different doctor.
- **Shop smart.** Always buy your herbal products from reputable manufacturers and retailers. Remember that you can't count on the government to make sure that the products you're buying are safe and effective.
- **Follow the rules.** Always obey the manufacturer's guidelines for dosage. Read the label each time you buy a new supplement, and remember that products can vary widely in concentration. If you can't find the information on the bottle, look it up.
- **Choose your battles wisely.** Don't use an herbal remedy when you need the potency of a pharmaceutical. If you've got an active bacterial infection, get the antibiotics. If you're in agony, get the prescription painkillers. Herbal remedies are effective, but they're almost always less potent than pharmaceutical drugs.
- **Don't forget . . .** that medicinal agents lurk in many places. For example, alcohol counts as a sedative, so don't drink if you're taking an herb or medication with sedating properties. Coffee is a stimulant, garlic is an anticlotting agent, and tea can have diuretic properties.

CHAPTER 18

Putting Herbs to Work

Herbs are available today in myriad forms, from fragrant bunches of flowers and leaves to tiny, uniform
tablets sealed into plastic bottles. All those choices
can be exciting—or unsettling—and many consumers are no doubt missing out on the benefits of
herbs because they simply don't know what to make
of them. They also might be unsure of the safe use
of herbal remedies: how to take them, how much to
take, and where to go for help if they need it.

How Herbs Are Sold

Herbs can be bought—and used—in many different forms. They're sold individually or in combination formulas, in topical or oral preparations, processed and packaged or *au naturel*.

- **Bulk herbs.** This is the plant at its most natural (unless you count the way it was when it was still growing). Bulk, or crude, herbs are the medicinal or therapeutic parts of a plant that have been harvested and separated from the nontherapeutic parts.

- **Powdered herbs.** These herbs have been dried and ground up. They can be used to make teas, poured into capsules, or taken straight.

- **Teas: Infusions and decoctions.** A tea or decoction is made by drawing the herb's constituents—its pigments, essential oils, nutrients, and phytochemicals—into water, which acts as a solvent to dissolve the plant matter (a tea is steeped, a decoction is boiled). Leaves and flowers are generally made into infusions, and roots and bark are made into decoctions.

- **Tinctures.** A tincture is an herbal extraction that uses a chemical solution (most often alcohol) as the solvent. Tinctures are stronger than crude or powdered herbs and teas/decoctions, and are easy to take (they're also readily absorbed into your bloodstream).

- **Extracts.** Herbal extracts are sold as liquids or solids (capsules or tablets) and are also easy to use.

- **Essential oils.** These are highly concentrated oils—not thick or greasy, but watery and volatile. Essential oils are plant extracts that contain only the "essential" ingredients: the plant's phytochemicals and its fragrance. Used in aromatherapy, essential oils are either inhaled or applied directly to the skin (usually after being diluted in a *carrier* oil, such as almond or sesame oil). They're also incorporated into topical herbal treatments such as lotions and creams.

- **Topical treatments.** These include ointments (salves), gels, lotions, infused oils, and creams, and can contain wildly varying amounts of herbs. Some have a medicinal or therapeutic dose of something—enough calendula (*Calendula officinalis*) to relieve your rash, for example—while others have just enough to make the product smell nice.

Many Considerations

Choosing and using herbal remedies shouldn't be an ordeal, and it shouldn't require a degree in botany or medicine (or both). But there are a few important issues to consider.

Consider potency: Some herbs can do their work at their natural concentration: Flaxseed (*Linum usitatissimum*), for example, can be used straight. Other herbs need to be concentrated.

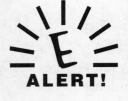
ALERT!

Among the various remedies taken internally, teas have the least potency—and therefore the least medicinal effect. Tinctures are a bit more powerful than teas, extracts are more powerful than tinctures, and concentrated extracts are the most potent.

For example, a handful of ginkgo (*Ginkgo biloba*) leaves won't do much for you on its own, as it takes several pounds of natural ginkgo to make a dose of real therapeutic value.

An herbal product that's been standardized is guaranteed to contain a certain amount of one or more specific compounds, which have been identified as the active, or therapeutic, ingredients. Herbalists agree that the best standardized extracts, at least as far as herbal medicine is concerned, are made from crude (whole plant) extracts, not isolated constituents. Thus, the label will read "Grape Seed Extract with Resveratrol" and not "Resveratrol" or "Antioxidant Complex." Herbs that are typically sold as standardized extracts include:

- Bilberry (*Vaccinium myrtillus*)
- Garlic (*Allium sativum*)
- Ginkgo (*Ginkgo biloba*)
- Grape (*Vitis vinifera*)
- Hawthorn (*Crataegus monogyna, C. oxyacantha*)
- Kava (*Piper methysticum*)
- Milk thistle (*Silybum marianum*)
- Saw palmetto (*Serenoa repens*)
- Saint John's wort (*Hypericum perforatum*)

Know What the Pros Know

Unlike pharmaceutical preparations, which typically offer very limited choices (will that be gelcaps or caplets?) or a single, one-size-fits-all formulation, herbs give you a variety of options. Here's how to navigate them:

Buying in Bulk

Buying bulk herbs is a much more tactile experience than buying ready-made remedies. It also gives you a chance to see exactly what you're getting. If you have a choice between fresh and dried, herbalists recommend the fresh in most cases.

When you're buying bulk herbs, be sure to give them a sniff first. Every herb will smell like something, even if it's just grass.

Not every herb smells like rose petals—and plenty of them don't. Chamomile (*Matricaria recutita*) and lavender (*Lavandula angustifolia*) have a pleasant floral fragrance, and peppermint (*Mentha x piperita*) and rosemary (*Rosmarinus officinalis*) smell sharp and appealing. But sage (*Salvia officinalis, S. lavandulaefolia*) has a musty-old-attic odor, and valerian (*Valeriana officinalis*) is reminiscent of an old pair of socks.

If you're buying dried herbs, remember that an herb that's fragrant when it's fresh should be fragrant when it's dried, too. Herbs that are colorful while they're growing should be colorful in the store (and dried herbs should retain much of the color they had when fresh).

Tincture How-To's

Most tinctures are made with alcohol, but alcohol-free products made with glycerin are also available. A tincture's concentration will be listed as a ratio: The first number indicates the amount of herb (this will be a 1), and the second indicates the amount of solution. Many tinctures contain one part herb and five parts solution, and so have a ratio of 1:5. The smaller the second number, the stronger the remedy will be.

Buying Herbal Extracts

Herbal extracts are sold as liquids or solids (capsules and tablets) and can be anywhere from 1 to 100 times more concentrated than crude herbs. The concept works like the one used for tinctures, but it's explained differently: The first number indicates the concentration, the second represents the herb in its natural state (it's always a 1). The bigger the first number is, the stronger the preparation will be.

ALERT!

Don't confuse herbal potency formulas with the one used in homeopathy, which works in the opposite direction: The more a remedy is diluted, the more potent it is believed to be. Homeopathic remedies are classified according to the number of times they're diluted (the more dilutions, the stronger the remedy), so a 12C or 12X remedy will be stronger than a 6C or 6X (homeopathy also uses a few different potency scales).

For example, an extract that's four times as strong as the crude herb has a ratio of 4:1. Fluid extracts are often sold in a 1:1 potency, meaning they're not concentrated.

Advice on Storing

Different herbs and herbal preparations have different considerations, but almost all should be stored the same way: in dark-colored, airtight glass containers kept in a cool, dry place. Herbs can quickly degrade and lose their medicinal muscle when exposed to even small amounts of sunlight and oxygen.

Every herb has its own lifespan, but, generally speaking, you can keep fresh herbs until they get slimy (or until you dry them). Dried herbs will generally keep about a year when stored correctly.

Powdered herbs generally keep just a few months before losing effectiveness. A tincture should be kept in its original container (most likely a dark-colored glass bottle with a dropper top). Stored correctly, tinctures will keep up to two years.

Both dried and liquid herbal extracts should keep about a year. Essential oils will keep indefinitely. Many commercial lotions and potions contain chemical preservatives, which give them the shelf life of a Twinkie (read: forever). But truly natural products contain natural preservatives, such as vitamin E, which don't last as long.

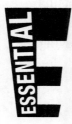

There's no official definition of "natural" when it comes to any consumer goods, including herbal products. For example, many cosmetics manufacturers use completely synthetic ingredients like caprylic acid or cetyl alcohol but list them on the label as being "derived from coconut oil." The only way to be sure a product is natural is to make it yourself.

Generally speaking, you can keep a product that doesn't contain synthetic preservatives for a few months—or until it changes consistency or starts to smell funny. Keeping it in the refrigerator should extend its life. Always check the expiration date on any packaged herbal product.

Smart Shopping

Health food stores and herbal shops are usually friendly places, but it can be daunting to face row after row of unfamiliar things. Here are a few rules to live (and shop) by:

Buy the Right Herb

Sounds obvious, but many plants have similar names, and buying the wrong one is easier than it sounds. For example, "danshen" sounds a lot like "dang shen," but danshen (*Salvia miltiorrhiza*) is used to treat cardiovascular disease, while dang shen (*Codonopsis pilosula*) is an immune tonic and energy booster. To make things worse, some people spell "dang shen" as "dangshen." Be sure you know both the common and botanical name of the plant you're buying.

Buy the Right Part(s)

Some herbs contain several active compounds that deliver very different actions—and these chemicals are found if different parts of the plant. For example, the gel and juice of the aloe (*Aloe vera*) plant contain several anti-inflammatory chemicals, which can treat burns (externally) and ulcers (internally). But the latex (the milky sap contained in the rind) contains anthraquinones, which work as a potent stimulant laxative. Thus, unless you're looking for constipation relief, be sure the aloe product you're buying is made from the gel, not the latex.

Buy the Right Preparation

Some herbs are effective medicines when used externally—but dangerous toxins when ingested. Both arnica (*Arnica montana*) and comfrey (*Symphytum officinale*), for example, can treat bruises and muscle aches and are used in a variety of creams, ointments, and other topical treatments. But taken internally, each can cause serious problems (arnica is toxic to the heart, comfrey to the liver). Arnica is used internally in homeopathic remedies (see Chapter 1), but they are extremely dilute and so are completely nontoxic.

Herbs are classified as either wild-grown or farm-grown. Wild-grown herbs, as the name implies, grew on their own and were harvested by people in a process called *wildcrafting*. Farm-grown herbs were produced commercially.

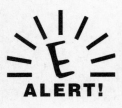

ALERT!

Some popular medicinal plants, including American ginseng (*Panax quinquefolius*), echinacea (*Echinacea purpurea*), goldenseal (*Hydrastis canadensis*), and kava (*Piper methysticum*) are threatened or endangered in the wild. Avoid buying them as wildcrafted herbs or products and always buy from a reputable manufacturer, ideally one that uses organically grown herbs.

Most people like the idea of using plants that grew naturally, unfettered by humans and all of our issues. But wild-grown herbs may have been exposed to chemicals and pesticides (they may have grown beside a highway or near a polluted stream). In addition, some herbs are endangered in the wild, meaning they stand the best chance of survival if they're cultivated commercially.

The best choice is to buy organically grown herbs that were raised in the United States according to our organic standards. That means they were raised without conventional pesticides, artificial fertilizers, or sewage.

Working with a Professional

If you have a serious health concern or are interested in broadening your herbal acumen beyond the basics, find a professional: an herbalist, a natural medicine practitioner, or a conventional doctor who uses herbs. Many doctors who practice complementary and alternative medicine (CAM) incorporate herbs, and although not all are licensed in every state, you can probably find at least one type of practitioner in your area (see Appendix C for some suggestions).

Herbalists

In the United States, there's no official definition of an herbalist, and there's no licensing or certification system in place for them. However, the American Herbalists Guild awards certification to herbalists who have at least four years of training and clinical experience. A professional member of AHG is considered a registered herbalist (RH) and will have the designation "RH (AHG)" after his or her name.

Naturopathic Doctors

Naturopaths are fully accredited physicians who have attended a four-year residential medical school and passed a postdoctoral board exam. A naturopath will have the designation "ND"—for Naturopathic Doctor.

Right now, naturopaths are licensed in fifteen states: Alaska, Arizona, California, Connecticut, Hawaii, Idaho, Kansas, Maine, Minnesota (as of July 2009), Montana, New Hampshire, Oregon, Utah, Vermont, and Washington, plus the District of Columbia and the U.S. territories of Puerto Rico and the Virgin Islands.

Chiropractors

Chiropractors, also known as doctors of chiropractic or chiropractic physicians, primarily treat neuromuscular issues—problems in the muscles, bones, and nervous system—like recurrent back pain and headaches. Many incorporate nutritional therapy and herbal medicine into their practices.

Chiropractic is arguably the largest and best known of the CAM professions. There are more than 60,000 practicing chiropractors in the United States, and chiropractic is recognized and licensed in all fifty states. Licensed chiropractors have completed at least four years of professional study and have passed national board and state licensing exams.

Traditional Chinese Medicine Practitioners

Traditional Chinese Medicine (TCM) uses herbs to treat all kinds of conditions and illnesses, which are almost always tied to an imbalance in the body. In TCM, herbs are generally used in combination with other medicinals (which are most often herbs, but can be minerals or animal products). Many formulas contain as many as fifty different components.

TCM practitioners are licensed in forty-three states; states that don't recognize TCM practitioners are Alabama, Delaware, Kansas, Mississippi, North Dakota, Oklahoma, South Dakota, and Wyoming.

Depending on which state you're in, licensed practitioners might have a few different designations. For example, a practitioner in Arkansas will be identified as a "DOM," or Doctor of Oriental Medicine, while his counterpart in New Hampshire will be identified by the letters "LAc" or "Lic.Ac.," for Licensed Acupuncturist.

Ayurvedic Physicians

Ayurvedic practitioners use herbs as food as well as medicine; herbs are often incorporated into therapeutic massage and other types of bodywork.

According to the National Institutes of Health (NIH), less than half of 1 percent of Americans—only about 750,000 people—have ever used Ayurveda, in part because it can be tough to find a qualified practitioner.

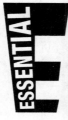

Some Ayurvedic practitioners working in the United States have training in naturopathic medicine, while others studied in India, where Ayurvedic training closely resembles that of U.S. medical schools and can take up to five years. In this country, Ayurvedic medicine is taught at a handful of private institutions.

Right now, there is no national standard for certification or training for Ayurvedic practitioners in the United States.

Ayurvedic practitioners sometimes use the title MD (Ayur.), which is the professional designation given in India. Practitioners who are accredited in the United States have the title DAv, or Diplomate in Ayurvedic Health Sciences, which is conferred by the American Ayurvedic Association.

Putting the Pieces Together

Putting herbs to work means understanding their uses—and limits—and deciding how to use them effectively.

In most cases, there are no ironclad rules when it comes to how much of an herbal remedy to take. All herbs are different, and remedies based on the same herb can vary enormously.

Experts determine what's known as a *therapeutic range* for medicines, with the smallest amount that would produce a benefit at one end and the maximum amount that the average person could take without experiencing unwanted effects at the other. Most herbs have a very wide range of efficacy, and it's nearly impossible to get a toxic dose of many of them. But while large doses of herbal remedies are usually safe, they're not necessary. The herbs that are in use today got here because they're effective—and practical.

Most manufacturers err on the cautious side when it comes to dosages, suggesting the lowest possible amount that you'd need to get the results you want.

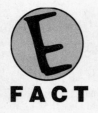

FACT

If you're using an alcohol-based tincture but are sensitive to alcohol, or if you're treating a child, you can get rid of a lot of it—not all, but a lot—by putting a small container of tincture into a pot of boiling water for a few minutes. This will allow the alcohol to evaporate.

When determining the best dose, you should always follow the manufacturer's guidelines. When you don't have any—the package doesn't have dosage information or you've made the remedy yourself—you can use these. For chronic conditions, adults should take the following doses:

- **Tea:** 3 to 4 cups a day
- **Tincture or syrup:** ½ to 1 teaspoon, three times a day

For acute problems, adults should take the following, until symptoms subside:

- **Tea:** ¼ to ½ cup every hour or two, up to three cups a day
- **Tincture or syrup:** ¼ to ½ teaspoon every 30 to 60 minutes

The dosages given here are for nonconcentrated products. Because commercial herbal extracts vary widely in their concentration, the best advice for taking a concentrated extract is to check the product's concentration level (see previous) and divide that by the dosages recommended here. Generally speaking, seniors should take a quarter of an adult dose. For chronic conditions, seniors should take the following doses:

- **Tea:** ½ to 1 cup, twice a day
- **Tincture or syrup:** ¼ to ½ teaspoon, twice a day

For acute problems, seniors should take the following, until symptoms subside:

- **Tea:** ⅛ to ¼ cup every hour or two, up to three cups a day
- **Tincture or syrup:** ⅛ to ¼ teaspoon every hour

Here are two formulas for determining the best dosage for a child:

- Take your child's age and add 12, then divide that number by the child's age. Then multiply the adult dosage by that number.
- Divide the child's age at his next birthday by 24.

Using these formulas, a six-year-old would get 30 percent of an adult dose, and a twelve-year-old would be given half. If you're treating a baby younger than six months (and you're breastfeeding), you can take the appropriate herb yourself—and pass it to your baby via your breastmilk.

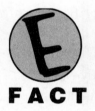

A recent study of health care professionals found that a full 79 percent of U.S. physicians and 82 percent of nurses say they recommend dietary supplements—including herbs—to their patients. A roughly equal number of doctors and nurses say they regularly use supplements themselves.

Practical Advice

Here is some advice on using herbs effectively:

- **Start slowly.** Take the smallest dose that's sensible, then see how you feel. Nothing? Take a bit more. Remember that herbs are almost always gentler and less potent than their pharmaceutical counterparts, so you don't want a dramatic reaction. If you're using an herb that can produce side effects you should exercise more restraint in increasing your dose than if you're using a more innocuous herb.

You also should be more careful about upping the dose if you're treating a senior or a child.

- **Know what you're doing.** Research the condition that you're treating, including the various treatment options—herbal and conventional—and the benefits of each.

- **Don't overdo it.** Adverse reactions from the herbal remedies used most often today are extremely rate, but they can happen—most often when an herb is overused. If you take too much for too long, you can have problems.

- **Be a patient patient.** Because herbs work subtly, they have what's known as a long onset of action. Unlike a pharmaceutical painkiller, for example, a dose of willow (*Salix alba*) won't get rid of your headache in a half an hour. And if you take psyllium (*Plantago ovata, P. psyllium*) to help relieve constipation, you'll have to wait longer than you would if you took a harsh pharmaceutical laxative.

- **Take the long view.** The general rule of thumb is to give an herbal remedy a few weeks before deciding if it's working or not. There are some exceptions to this rule: Some herbs work more quickly, but others take longer to produce results.

- **Don't use short-term remedies for long-term problems.** If you find yourself constantly reaching for the same type of acute remedy—a laxative to relieve constipation or an antacid to quell heartburn—it's time to change tactics. Contact a professional, who can help you address the underlying problem.

CHAPTER 19

Making Your Own Herbal Remedies

With only a few common tools and a few simple ingredients, which are available at most any herb shop or natural foods store, you can open your own phytopharmacy. And while it's arguably much easier and a lot less messy to buy your remedies ready-made, many people find that the do-it-yourself, get-your-hands-dirty approach is both rewarding and effective. By making your own remedies, you can control more aspects of the product you're using, and you'll gain a greater understanding of the power of plants.

Homemade Healing

Maybe you're the type of person who thinks everything's better when it's homemade. Maybe you love to cook and experiment with recipes. Or maybe there's just no decent herb shop in your town. Whatever the reason, you're ready to take the plunge into the world of home-based herbalism. Rosemary Gladstar, a leading herbalist and educator and director of the International Herb Symposium, offers the following suggestions—and recipes—to get you started.

Tools of the Trade

To make most herbal remedies, you'll need a short list of supplies. It includes:

- Big canning jars for storing herbs and making tinctures
- Cheesecloth or muslin, for straining herbal preparations
- A grater (for grating beeswax)
- A large, double-mesh, stainless steel strainer
- Measuring cups
- Nonaluminum cooking pots with tight-fitting lids

You might want to set aside a coffee grinder to use for grinding the tough spices like licorice (*Glycyrrhiza glabra*) root and cinnamon (*Cinnamomum verum, C. aromaticum*) bark that you'll use in your remedies. Just don't use the same grinder that you use for coffee—neither your remedies nor your morning cup of Joe will benefit from that blending of flavors.

You should keep your pantry stocked with a few of the staples that are used in many herbal remedies. They include:

- **Aloe** (*Aloe vera*) gel, for creams
- **Apricot** (*Prunus armeniaca*), almond (*Prunus dulcis*), and grape (*Vitis vinifera*) seed oils, for facial creams
- **Cocoa** (*Theobroma cacao*) butter, for infused oils and creams
- **Coconut** (*Cocos nucifera*) oil, for infused oils and creams
- **Honey**, for syrups
- **Lanolin**, for creams

- **Natural beeswax**, for ointments
- **Olive** (*Olea europaea*) oil, for infused oils and ointments
- **Sesame** (*Sesamum indicum*) oil, for infused oils

Here are a few things to keep in mind when making your own remedies:

- Herbs and herbal preparations do best when they're stored in air-tight glass jars, out of direct light, in a cool area. Light, oxygen, and heat can degrade them.
- Never use aluminum pots or containers—aluminum can react with the herbs. Stick to glass, ceramic, stainless steel, or cast iron.
- Store all remedies and ingredients—especially essential oils and alcohol-based tinctures—out of children's reach. Many essential oils are extremely toxic, even in very small doses.

Therapeutic Teas

A tea is, without question, the simplest of herbal remedies to prepare—and use. Even the most inept of homemakers can boil water, and that's really all it takes to make a cup of tea.

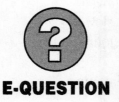

E-QUESTION

What makes tea?
Technically speaking, tea can mean only one thing: *Camellia sinensis*, either in its natural state or dried and mixed with boiling water to make an infusion of the same name. But many medicinal herbs, including rooibos (*Aspalathus linearis*) in South Africa and mate (*Ilex paraguariensis*) in South America, are regularly brewed up as "teas," to be enjoyed as beverages as well as therapeutic agents.

Herbal teas can be used for several purposes. First, herbal tea is a beverage, good for socializing and relaxing as well as hydrating. It's also useful as a topical herbal preparation for your skin as well as your hair.

Tea is an effective vehicle for administering the medicinal components of plants as well. Teas are aqueous (water) extractions of crude herbs or herbal powders. There are a few methods you can use: infusion, which is best for the delicate aerial parts (leaves and flowers), and decoction, which is used with tougher materials (like bark, seeds, and roots).

Making an Infusion

An infusion is what most people think of when they think tea: it's what you get when you soak a bunch of tea leaves in hot water.

To make a tea with loose herbs, put the plant material into a strainer and into a cup, then fill the cup with boiling water. Cover the cup: The medicinal value of many herbs, including peppermint (*Mentha x piperita*), is contained in the essential oils, so you'll want to keep the steam from escaping. You can also make an infusion using a French coffee press; just don't use the same one you use to make coffee.

When making tea, use about 1 teaspoon of dried herbs per cup of water. Steep for 15 minutes or longer. The more herb you use and the longer you let it steep, the stronger your tea will be.

Making a Decoction

Decoctions are the best way to get the medicinal constituents out of the tougher parts of the plant—like the roots and bark. To make one, put the herbs into a saucepan, add cold water, cover, and increase the heat slowly until it reaches a boil. Simmer the mixture for at least 15 minutes. The longer it simmers, the stronger it will be.

To make a decoction, you'll need about 1 teaspoon of the herbal mixture per cup of water.

Making Sun Tea

Add a bunch of dried herbs (leaves and flowers) to a large, clear glass container (use the same amounts recommended for infusions or extractions, above), cover tightly, and let it sit in the sun for several hours.

You'll know it's done when the water turns the same color it would if you were brewing tea via the infusion or decoction method.

Using Teas

You'll take a cup of most teas three or four times a day, or as needed. If you're treating a chronic condition, drink three or four cups a day for several weeks. For more on dosages, see Chapter 18.

Here are some therapeutic teas to try:

Constipation Tea

Ingredients:

3 parts fennel (*Foeniculum vulgare*) seed
1 part senna (*Cassia officinalis, Senna alexandrina*) leaf
½ part cascara sagrada (*Rhamnus purshiana*) root
1 part licorice (*Glycyrrhiza glabra*) root
½ part cinnamon (*Cinnamomum verum, C. aromaticum*) bark

If constipation persists after using this tea, try increasing the cascara sagrada to 1 part and the senna to 1½ parts.

Follow the directions above to make a decoction.

Sore Throat Soother

Ingredients:

2 parts licorice (*Glycyrrhiza glabra*) root
1 part cinnamon (*Cinnamomum verum, C. aromaticum*) bark
2 parts fennel (*Foeniculum vulgare*) seeds
2 parts echinacea (*Echinacea purpurea*) root
1 part marshmallow (*Althaea officinalis*) root
½ part orange (*Citrus sinensis*) peel

*If you can't find marshmallow root, you can substitute slipper elm (*Ulmus rubra*) bark.*

Follow the directions above to make a decoction.

Anti-insomnia Tea

Ingredients:

2 parts chamomile (*Matricaria recutita*) flowers

2 parts passionflower (*Passiflora incarnata*) leaves and flowers

2 parts lemon balm (*Melissa officinalis*) leaf

1 part valerian (*Valeriana officinalis*) root

½ part rose (*Rosa canina R. spp.*) hips

¼ part lavender (*Lavandula angustifolia*) flowers

Drink in the evening, at least an hour or two before bed (you don't want to wake up because you need to use the bathroom). If you want something stronger, you can make this formula into a tincture (see instructions on pages 260–261); take ¼ teaspoon of the tincture at bedtime.

Follow the directions for an infusion or sun tea, above.

Herbal Hair Tea

Combine equal parts of the following herbs (pick one condition to treat at a time):

Equal parts of nettle (*Urtica dioica*) and rosemary (*Rosmarinus officinale*) if you have an oily scalp. Rosemary and juniper (*Juniperus communis*) can help clear up dandruff. And nettle (*Urtica dioica*), rosemary (*Rosmarinus officinale*), and lavender (*Lavandula angustifolia*) make an effective remedy for hair loss. All of these can be made as infusions.

To give your hair color a boost, try an infusion of chamomile (*Matricaria recutita*) or calendula (*Calendula officinalis*) for blonde or highlighted hair or a decoction of black walnut (*Juglans nigra*) hulls for darker shades. Follow the directions, above. Apply to your hair after shampooing; don't rinse out.

To boost the effectiveness of the oily hair treatment, add a drop or two of rosemary (*Rosmarinus officinalis*) essential oil. Lavender (*Lavandula angustifolia*) essential oil will increase the effect of the dandruff and hair-loss teas.

Sweet-Tasting Syrups

Syrups are a great way to treat children with herbs. They're sweet and they go down much easier than other liquid remedies. If properly stored, syrups will last for several weeks.

To make an herbal syrup, first make a quart of an infusion (see page 256) and then simmer it down and mix with honey or another sweetener (like maple syrup or brown sugar). Note that experts advise against giving raw (unpasteurized) honey to children younger than a year because of the risk of botulism. If you're making syrup to give to a baby, you can replace honey with commercial maple syrup or brown sugar.

Adults should take ½ to 1 teaspoon three times a day for chronic conditions and ¼ to ½ teaspoon every 30 to 60 minutes, until symptoms improve, when treating an acute problem. Children and seniors should be given smaller doses (see Chapter 18).

Here are a few syrup recipes:

Cinnamon-Echinacea Cold Syrup

Ingredients:
1 part dried echinacea (*Echinacea purpurea*) root
1 part cinnamon (*Cinnamomum verum, C. aromaticum*) bark
½ part fresh ginger (*Zingiber officinalis*) root, grated or chopped

This is perfect for treating colds and flu—especially in kids.

1. Add 2 ounces (about 8 tablespoons) of the herb mixture to a quart of cold water. Bring to a boil, then simmer until the liquid is reduced by half (leave the lid slightly ajar).
2. Strain the herbs from the liquid and discard, then pour the liquid back into the pot.
3. Add 1 cup of honey (or another sweetener) and heat the mixture through.
4. Remove from heat, let cool, and transfer to glass bottles. Store in the refrigerator.

Heart-Healthy Hawthorn Syrup

Ingredients:

A handful of dried seedless hawthorn (*Crataegus monogyna, C. oxyacantha*) berries

Apple juice (enough to cover berries in pan)

Honey to taste

Ginger (*Zingiber officinalis*) to taste, grated or powdered

Cinnamon (*Cinnamomum verum, C. aromaticum*) to taste

This syrup incorporates hawthorn berries, which are rich in antioxidants and have proven cardiovascular benefits. If the berries have seeds in them, soak and press them through a sieve to remove the seeds before using.

1. Put the berries into a pan with just enough apple juice to cover them. Simmer over low heat for 15 minutes. Remove from heat and let stand overnight.
2. Season with honey, ginger, and cinnamon to taste.
3. Return to heat, add enough apple juice to create a syrupy consistency, and heat through.
4. Remove from heat, let cool, and transfer to glass bottles. Store in the refrigerator.

Tinctures

Tinctures are liquid herbal extracts made by combining the herbs with a solvent. Traditional tinctures are made with alcohol, but you can also use vinegar or vegetable glycerin (available at many health food stores) instead. Tinctures are typically more potent than infusions, decoctions, or syrups.

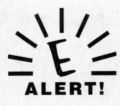

When you're making tinctures at home, never use industrial alcohols, such as rubbing alcohol (isopropyl alcohol) or methylated spirits (methyl alcohol). Both are extremely toxic. Stick to beverage alcohols, such as vodka and brandy, or use a nonalcoholic substitute like glycerin.

Start with bulk herbs (fresh is best) and chop them finely. Put them into a clean glass jar and add enough alcohol—80- or 100-proof vodka, gin, or brandy—to cover them with about 2 or 3 inches of fluid. Cover with a tight-fitting lid, place the jar in a warm, dark spot, and leave it there for four to six weeks—the longer, the better.

Once a day, shake the jar to keep the herbs from settling at the bottom.

When the time is up, strain the herbs and discard them. Transfer the tincture to a small glass bottle (ideally one with a dropper, which makes it easier to get the right dose). Stored properly, it will keep for two years or longer. Be sure to keep tinctures out of the reach of children.

Brain-Boosting Tincture

Ingredients:

2 parts ginkgo (*Ginkgo biloba*) leaves

2 parts gotu kola (*Centella asiatica*) leaves

1 part peppermint (*Mentha x piperita*) leaves and flowers

1 part rosemary (*Rosmarinus officinale*)

Take 1 teaspoon of tincture 2 to 3 times daily for at least three weeks. This tincture really does work at increasing memory, but you'll need to take it for several weeks before you'll notice a difference.

Follow the directions for making a tincture, above.

Headache Relief Tincture

Ingredients:

1 part California poppy (*Eschscholzia californica*) seeds

1 part feverfew (*Tanacetum parthenium*) leaves and flowers

1 part lavender (*Lavandula angustifolia*) flowers

Keep this relaxing, pain-fighting combination on hand for whenever headaches strike.

Follow the directions for making a tincture, above.

Infused Oils and Ointments

Herbal oils can be used alone or as a base for creams or ointments. There are two ways to make infused oils: using the sun or using the stove. You can use many types of vegetable oil as your base—coconut (*Cocos nucifera*) and almond (*Prunus dulcis*) are popular choices—and add an equal amount of cocoa (*Theobroma cacao*) butter to thicken the mixture, if you like (this works best with the stovetop method).

Making Solar-Infused Oils

Place a handful of dried herbs into a clean, clear glass jar and fill the jar with oil (you'll use about 2 ounces, or 8 tablespoons, of herbs per pint of oil). Cover tightly and place in a warm sunny spot. Leave it there for two weeks. When the time is up, pour the mixture through a piece of cheesecloth or muslin, making sure to wring the cloth tightly and catch every last drop of oil.

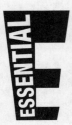

When making infused oils, you'll get the best results with dried herbs. Plant material that contains too much moisture can cause the oil to get moldy. (Your oil can also grow mold if it's made or stored in a jar with an ill-fitting lid, which can allow moisture to get in.)

Discard the herbs and replace them with a new batch, then let the oil and herbs steep for another two weeks. Transfer to clean glass bottles. Stored correctly, infused oils will last several months.

The Stovetop Method

If you don't have a lot of sunshine (or a month to wait), you can make your oil on the stove using a double boiler. Put the herbs and oil into the top section, fill the bottom with water, and bring it to a low boil. Let the oil simmer gently for 30 to 60 minutes, checking frequently to make sure the oil isn't overheating (it will start to smoke if that's the case). The lower and longer you let it simmer, the better your oil will be.

Here's one recipe to try:

Calming Massage Oil

Ingredients:

1 part coconut (*Cocos nucifera*) oil

1 part almond (*Prunus dulcis*) oil

1 part cocoa (*Theobroma cacao*) butter

1 part chamomile (*Matricaria recutita*) flowers

1 part lavender (*Lavandula angustifolia*) leaves

1 part lemon balm (*Melissa officinalis*) leaves and flowers

This infusion contains three tried-and-true herbal relaxants, plus three soothing and moisturizing plant oils.

Prepare according to the instructions, above.

Making Herbal Ointments

Ointments, also known as salves, are thick, oil-based preparations used to treat superficial wounds (like scrapes, burns, and insect bites) and soothe aching muscles and joints. Here's how to make them:

1. Start with an infused oil (see above) that's been strained. Put the oil into a small pan and add grated beeswax—¼ cup per cup of infused oil. Heat on low, until the beeswax is completely melted, then remove from the heat.
2. Test a small amount for consistency by putting it into the freezer for a minute or two to cool it. If it seems too hard (you can't spread it easily), heat it again and add more oil. If it's too oily, reheat and add more beeswax.
3. When you've got the consistency you want, transfer the ointment to clean glass jars. Stored properly, ointments will last several months.

Try this recipe:

Burn (and Baby Bottom) Ointment

Ingredients:
1 part calendula (*Calendula officinalis*) flowers
1 part comfrey (*Symphytum officinale*) leaves
1 part comfrey (*Symphytum officinale*) root
1 part Saint John's wort (*Hypericum perforatum*) flowers
1 part olive (*Olea europaea*) oil
Beeswax, grated

This is a classic remedy that combines skin-soothing, inflammation-fighting and germ-killing herbs.

Follow the instructions for making an herbal ointment, above.

Beauty Blends

Herbs make a great addition to your personal care routine and can be incorporated into toners and astringents, moisturizers, and powders.

Making Astringent Solutions

Herbs with astringent, or drying, properties can be used to cleanse and refresh the skin and to gently remove excess oil. Here's how to make one:

1. Pack a wide-mouthed glass jar with dried herbs, leaving a few inches of space at the top.
2. Fill the jar with alcohol (or another solvent) so that there's an inch or two of fluid above the top of the herbs. Cover tightly.
3. Put the jar in a warm place and leave it there for 3 or 4 weeks.
4. When the time is up, strain the herbs and discard them. Transfer the liquid to a smaller bottle.

Here's a recipe to try at home:

Bay Rum Aftershave and Astringent

Ingredients:
1 part bay (*Laurus nobilis*) leaves (fresh if possible)
1 part cloves (*Syzygium aromaticum*), whole
1 part ginger (*Zingiber officinalis*), fresh (grated) or ground
Optional: Ground allspice (*Pimenta dioica*) to give your lotion a spicier scent

This preparation works equally well as an aftershave and facial astringent.

Follow the instructions for making an astringent, above.

Making Facial Creams

Facial creams are emulsions, or mixtures of oil and water. Do-it-yourself herbal creams typically contain aqueous ingredients such as distilled water and/or aloe (*Aloe vera*) gel or a water-based herbal infusion, plus vegetable oils—you can use apricot (*Prunus armeniaca*), almond (*Prunus dulcis*), or grape (*Vitis vinifera*) seed oils or an herb-infused oil (see above). They also might contain essential oils, which impart a scent and treat specific skin conditions. Some of the most popular essential oils used in facial products include rose (*Rosa damascena*), chamomile (*Matricaria recutita*), lavender (*Lavandula angustifolia*), and calendula (*Calendula officinalis*).

Some facial creams also contains essential oils. Use one of the following, based on your skin type:

- **Lavender** (*Lavandula angustifolia*)   for all skin types
- **Chamomile** (*Matricaria recutita*)   for sensitive skin
- **Grapefruit** (*Citrus paradisi*)   for oily skin
- **Rose** (*Rosa damascena*)   also known as damask rose, rose otto, or Bulgarian rose, for all skin types, especially dry and/or sensitive

Here's a cream to try:

Rosemary's Famous Facial Cream

Ingredients:
⅔ cup distilled water
⅓ cup aloe (*Aloe vera*) gel
1 or 2 drops of essential oil (see above)
¾ cup apricot (*Prunus armeniaca*) oil
⅓ cup coconut (*Cocos nucifera)* oil or cocoa (*Theobroma cacao*) butter
¼ teaspoon lanolin
½ to 1 ounce beeswax, grated

Expert herbalist Rosemary Gladstar has been making this cream for over thirty years (it's a staple in her correspondence course, "The Science and Art of Herbalism"). It rivals any department-store concoction and works as both an emollient (softening agent) and humectant (it helps the skin retain moisture).

1. Combine the distilled water, aloe gel, and essential oils in a glass cup or bowl, and set aside.
2. In a double boiler over low heat, combine the apricot oil, coconut oil (or cocoa butter), lanolin, and beeswax, and heat them just enough to melt the beeswax. Remove from heat.
3. Pour the oil mixture into a blender and allow it to cool completely. When it's room temperature, turn the blender on to its highest speed and add the water mixture, pouring as slowly as you can, to the oils. Don't pour the whole amount at once—watch the mixture closely, and when it looks thick and white, stop adding water.
4. Pour the cream into glass jars. Store in a cool location.

Common Health Concerns

Acid Indigestion (Dyspepsia)
- Artichoke (*Cynara cardunculus, C. scolymus*)
- Chamomile (*Matricaria recutita*)
- Lavender (*Lavandula angustifolia*)
- Licorice (*Glycyrrhiza glabra*)
- Peppermint (*Mentha x piperita*)
- Pineapple (*Ananas comosus*)
- Rosemary (*Rosmarinus officinalis*)
- Turmeric (*Curcuma longa*)

Acne
- Calendula (*Calendula officinalis*)
- Guggul (*Commiphora wightii, C. mukul*)
- Juniper (*Juniperus communis*)
- Red clover (*Trifolium pratense*)
- Tea tree (*Melaleuca alternifolia*)

Addictions and Alcoholism
- Danshen (*Salvia miltiorrhiza*)
- Ginkgo (*Ginkgo biloba*)
- Kudzu (*Pueraria lobata*)
- Passionflower (*Passiflora incarnata*)
- Saint John's wort (*Hypericum perforatum*)

Age-Related Cognitive Decline
- Cocoa (*Theobroma cacao*)
- Garlic (*Allium sativum*)
- Ginkgo (*Ginkgo biloba*)
- Grape (*Vitis vinifera*)
- Rooibos (*Aspalathus linearis*)

Age-Related Eye Disease
- Bilberry (*Vaccinium myrtillus*)
- Flax (*Linum usitatissimum*)
- Ginkgo (*Ginkgo biloba*)
- Grape (*Vitis vinifera*)
- Maritime pine (*Pinus pinaster*)

Aging Skin
- Coffee (*Coffea arabica*)
- Evening primrose (*Oenothera biennis*)
- Gotu kola (*Centella asiatica*)
- Grape (*Vitis vinifera*)
- Maritime pine (*Pinus pinaster*)
- Pineapple (*Ananas comosus*)
- Pomegranate (*Punica granatum*)
- Rose (*Rosa damascena, R. canina, R. spp.*)
- Tea (*Camellia sinensis*)

Allergies
- Butterbur (*Petasites hybridus*)
- Echinacea (*Echinacea purpurea*)
- Hops (*Humulus lupulus*)
- Licorice (*Glycyrrhiza glabra*)
- Nettle (*Urtica dioica*)
- Rooibos (*Aspalathus linearis*)
- Tea (*Camellia sinensis*)
- Tinospora (*Tinospora cordifolia*)
- Witch hazel (*Hamamelis virginiana*)

Altitude Sickness
- Asian ginseng (*Panax ginseng*)
- Ginkgo (*Ginkgo biloba*)
- Reishi (*Ganoderma lucidum*)

Alzheimer's Disease and Dementia
- Garlic (*Allium sativum*)
- Ginkgo (*Ginkgo biloba*)
- Grape (*Vitis vinifera*)
- Lemon balm (*Melissa officinalis*)
- Rooibos (*Aspalathus linearis*)
- Sage (*Salvia officinalis, S. lavandulaefolia*)
- Turmeric (*Curcuma longa*)

Anxiety
- Ashwagandha (*Withania somnifera*)
- Boswellia (*Boswellia serrata*)
- Chamomile (*Matricaria recutita*)
- Hops (*Humulus lupulus*)
- Kava (*Piper methysticum*)
- Lavender (*Lavandula angustifolia*)
- Lemon balm (*Melissa officinalis*)
- Passionflower (*Passiflora incarnata*)
- Valerian (*Valeriana officinalis*)

Arthritis (Osteoarthritis)
- Ashwagandha (*Withania somnifera*)
- Boswellia (*Boswellia serrata*)
- Camphor (*Cinnamomum camphora*)
- Cat's claw (*Uncaria guianensis, U. tomentosa*)
- Cayenne (*Capsicum annuum, C. frutescens*)
- Devil's claw (*Harpagphytum procumbens*)
- Ginger (*Zingiber officinale*)
- Guggul (*Commiphora wightii, C. mukul*)
- Nettle (*Urtica dioica*)
- Pineapple (*Ananas comosus*)
- Turmeric (*Curcuma longa*)

Asthma

- Boswellia (*Boswellia serrata*)
- Coffee (*Coffea arabica*)
- Eucalyptus (*Eucalyptus globulus*)
- Ginkgo (*Ginkgo biloba*)
- Grapefruit (*Citrus paradisi*)
- Guarana (*Paullinia cupana*)
- Maritime pine (*Pinus pinaster*)
- Tea (*Camellia sinensis*)

Athlete's Foot

- Camphor (*Cinnamomum camphora*)
- Clove (*Syzygium aromaticum*)
- Echinacea (*Echinacea purpurea*)
- Garlic (*Allium sativum*)
- Lavender (*Lavandula angustifolia*)
- Tea tree (*Melaleuca alternifolia*)

Athletic Performance

- American ginseng (*Panax quinquefolius*)
- Asian ginseng (*Panax ginseng*)
- Coffee (*Coffea arabica*)
- Cordyceps (*Cordyceps sinensis*)
- Eleuthero (*Eleutherococcus senticosus*)
- Guarana (*Paullinia cupana*)
- Maritime pine (*Pinus pinaster*)

Atopic Dermatitis

- Aloe (*Aloe vera*)
- Astragalus (*Astragalus membranaceus*)
- Hops (*Humulus lupulus*)
- Oats (*Avena sativa*)
- Rice bran (*Oryza sativa*)

Attention Deficit Hyperactivity Disorder (ADHD)

- Flax (*Linum usitatissimum*)
- Ginkgo (*Ginkgo biloba*)
- Maritime pine (*Pinus pinaster*)

Autoimmune Disorders

- Ashwagandha (*Withania somnifera*)
- Asian ginseng (*Panax ginseng*)
- Astragalus (*Astragalus membranaceus*)
- Bilberry (*Vaccinium myrtillus*)
- Feverfew (*Tanacetum parthenium*)
- Flax (*Linum usitatissimum*)
- Ginger (*Zingiber officinale*)
- Grape (*Vitis vinifera*)
- Licorice (*Glycyrrhiza glabra*)

Back Pain

- Cramp bark (*Viburnum opulus*)
- Devil's claw (*Harpagphytum procumbens*)
- Ginger (*Zingiber officinale*)
- Lavender (*Lavandula angustifolia*)
- Willow (*Salix alba*)

Bacterial Infection

- Aloe (*Aloe vera*)
- Barberry (*Berberis vulgaris*)
- Cat's claw (*Uncaria guianensis, U. tomentosa*)
- Clove (*Syzygium aromaticum*)
- Garlic (*Allium sativum*)
- Goldenseal (*Hydrastis canadensis*)
- Gotu kola (*Centella asiatica*)
- Saint John's wort (*Hypericum perforatum*)
- Tea tree (*Melaleuca alternifolia*)
- Tulsi (*Ocimum tenuiflorum, O. sanctum*)
- Witch hazel (*Hamamelis virginiana*)

Benign Prostatic Hyperplasia (BPH)

- Nettle (*Urtica dioica*)
- Saw palmetto (*Serenoa repens*)

Bloating and Water Retention

- Alfalfa (*Medicago sativa*)
- Dandelion (*Taraxacum officinale*)
- Juniper (*Juniperus communis*)
- Nettle (*Urtica dioica*)
- Tea (*Camellia sinensis*)

Breast Pain (Mastaglia)

- Evening primrose (*Oenothera biennis*)
- Red clover (*Trifolium pratense*)
- Vitex (*Vitex agnus-castus*)

Bruises

- Arnica (*Arnica montana*)
- Comfrey (*Symphytum officinale*)

Burns

- Aloe (*Aloe vera*)
- Calendula (*Calendula officinalis*)
- Camphor (*Cinnamomum camphora*)
- Lavender (*Lavandula angustifolia*)
- Marshmallow (*Althaea officinalis*)
- Saint John's wort (*Hypericum perforatum*)
- Tea tree (*Melaleuca alternifolia*)
- Witch hazel (*Hamamelis virginiana*)

Cancer

- Astragalus (*Astragalus membranaceus*)
- Cordyceps (*Cordyceps sinensis*)
- Evening primrose (*Oenothera biennis*)
- Ginger (*Zingiber officinale*)
- Grape (*Vitis vinifera*)
- Reishi (*Ganoderma lucidum*)
- Saw palmetto (*Serenoa repens*)
- Turmeric (*Curcuma longa*)

Canker Sores

- Calendula (*Calendula officinalis*)
- Clove (*Syzygium aromaticum*)
- Slippery elm (*Ulmus rubra*)
- Tea tree (*Melaleuca alternifolia*)

Cardiovascular Disease
- Danshen (*Salvia miltiorrhiza*)
- Grape (*Vitis vinifera*)
- Hawthorn (*Crataegus monogyna, C. oxyacantha*)
- Pomegranate (*Punica granatum*)

Cataracts
See Age-Related Eye Disease

Chronic Fatigue Syndrome
See Autoimmune Disorders

Cognitive Function and Memory
- Ginkgo (*Ginkgo biloba*)
- Sage (*Salvia officinalis, S. lavandulaefolia*)
- Schisandra (*Schisandra chinensis*)

Chronic Fatigue Syndrome
- Ashwagandha (*Withania somnifera*)
- Asian ginseng (*Panax ginseng*)
- Bilberry (*Vaccinium myrtillus*)

Chronic Venous Insufficiency
- Grape (*Vitis vinifera*)
- Horse chestnut (*Aesculus hippocastanum*)
- Maritime pine (*Pinus pinaster*)

Colds and Flu
- Andrographis (*Andrographis paniculata*)
- Echinacea (*Echinacea purpurea*)
- Elderberry (*Sambucus nigra*)
- Eucalyptus (*Eucalyptus globulus*)
- Garlic (*Allium sativum*)
- Ginger (*Zingiber officinale*)
- Licorice (*Glycyrrhiza glabra*)
- Peppermint (*Mentha x piperita*)

Cold Sores
- Aloe (*Aloe vera*)
- Clove (*Syzygium aromaticum*)
- Echinacea (*Echinacea purpurea*)
- Garlic (*Allium sativum*)
- Lemon balm (*Melissa officinalis*)
- Licorice (*Glycyrrhiza glabra*)
- Sage (*Salvia officinalis, S. lavandulaefolia*)
- Saint John's wort (*Hypericum perforatum*)

Constipation
- Aloe (*Aloe vera*)
- Fenugreek (*Trigonella foenum-graecum*)
- Flax (*Linum usitatissimum*)
- Konjac (*Amorphophallus konjac, A. rivieri*)
- Olive (*Olea europaea*)
- Psyllium (*Plantago ovata, P. psyllium*)

Cough and Sore Throat
- Eucalyptus (*Eucalyptus globulus*)
- Ginger (*Zingiber officinale*)
- Marshmallow (*Althaea officinalis*)
- Slippery elm (*Ulmus rubra*)

Crohn's Disease
See Inflammatory Bowel Disease

Cuts and Scrapes
- Barberry (*Berberis vulgaris*)
- Calendula (*Calendula officinalis*)
- Eucalyptus (*Eucalyptus globulus*)
- Garlic (*Allium sativum*)
- Gotu kola (*Centella asiatica*)
- Horsetail (*Equisetum arvense*)
- Marshmallow (*Althaea officinalis*)
- Tea tree (*Melaleuca alternifolia*)
- Witch hazel (*Hamamelis virginiana*)
- Yarrow (*Achillea millefolium*)

Dandruff
- Juniper (*Juniperus communis*)
- Licorice (*Glycyrrhiza glabra*)
- Peppermint (*Mentha x piperita*)
- Tea (*Camellia sinensis*)
- Tea tree (*Melaleuca alternifolia*)

Deodorant
- Camphor (*Cinnamomum camphora*)
- Juniper (*Juniperus communis*)
- Rosemary (*Rosmarinus officinalis*)
- Sage (*Salvia officinalis, S. lavandulaefolia*)
- Tea tree (*Melaleuca alternifolia*)
- Yarrow (*Achillea millefolium*)

Depression
- Boswellia (*Boswellia serrata*)
- Lemon balm (*Melissa officinalis*)
- Rhodiola (*Rhodiola rosea*)
- Saint John's wort (*Hypericum perforatum*)

Dermatitis
See Inflammatory Skin Disorders

Diabetes
- Fenugreek (*Trigonella foenum-graecum*)
- Gymnema (*Gymnema sylvestre*)
- Konjac (*Amorphophallus konjac, A. rivieri*)
- Milk thistle (*Silybum marianum*)
- Psyllium (*Plantago ovata, P. psyllium*)
- Tulsi (*Ocimum tenuiflorum, O. sanctum*)

Diabetic Retinopathy
See Age-Related Eye Disease

Diaper Rash
- Calendula (*Calendula officinalis*)
- Lavender (*Lavandula angustifolia*)

Diarrhea

- Barberry (*Berberis vulgaris*)
- Juniper (*Juniperus communis*)
- Marshmallow (*Althaea officinalis*)
- Psyllium (*Plantago ovata, P. psyllium*)
- Sangre de grado (*Croton lechleri*)
- Tea (*Camellia sinensis*)

Digestion Support

- Chamomile (*Matricaria recutita*)
- Cinnamon (*Cinnamomum verum, C. aromaticum*)
- Fennel (*Foeniculum vulgare*)
- Garlic (*Allium sativum*)
- Hops (*Humulus lupulus*)
- Lavender (*Lavandula angustifolia*)
- Oats (*Avena sativa*)
- Peppermint (*Mentha x piperita*)
- Pineapple (*Ananas comosus*)

Disease Prevention

- Garlic (*Allium sativum*)
- Grape (*Vitis vinifera*)
- Oats (*Avena sativa*)
- Olive (*Olea europaea*)
- Pomegranate (*Punica granatum*)
- Rose (*Rosa canina, R. spp.*)
- Soy (*Glycine max*)
- Tea (*Camellia sinensis*)

Dry Hair and Scalp

- Flax (*Linum usitatissimum*)
- Jojoba (*Simmondsia chinensis*)
- Olive (*Olea europaea*)

Dry Skin

- Borage (*Borago officinalis*)
- Cocoa (*Theobroma cacao*)
- Evening primrose (*Oenothera biennis*)
- Flax (*Linum usitatissimum*)
- Jojoba (*Simmondsia chinensis*)
- Olive (*Olea europaea*)

Ear Infection

- Garlic (*Allium sativum*)
- Goldenseal (*Hydrastis canadensis*)
- Lavender (*Lavandula angustifolia*)
- Saint John's wort (*Hypericum perforatum*)
- Witch hazel (*Hamamelis virginiana*)

Eczema

See Inflammatory Skin Disorders

Erectile Dysfunction

See Sexual Dysfunction (Male)

Fibromyalgia

See Autoimmune Disorders

Foodborne Illness (Food Poisoning)

- Ginger (*Zingiber officinale*)
- Juniper (*Juniperus communis*)
- Sangre de grado (*Croton lechleri*)

Gas and Flatulence

- Alfalfa (*Medicago sativa*)
- Artichoke (*Cynara cardunculus, C. scolymus*)
- Fennel (*Foeniculum vulgare*)
- Lavender (*Lavandula angustifolia*)
- Peppermint (*Mentha x piperita*)

Glaucoma

See Age-Related Eye Disease

Hair Care

- Amla (*Emblica officinalis, Phyllanthus emblica*)
- Eclipta (*Eclipta alba, E. prostrata*)
- Horsetail (*Equisetum arvense*)
- Marshmallow (*Althaea officinalis*)
- Nettle (*Urtica dioica*)
- Psyllium (*Plantago ovata, P. psyllium*)
- Tea (*Camellia sinensis*)

Hair Color

- Amla (*Emblica officinalis, Phyllanthus emblica*)
- Chamomile (*Matricaria recutita*)
- Eclipta (*Eclipta alba, E. prostrata*)
- Tea (*Camellia sinensis*)

Hair Loss

- Eclipta (*Eclipta alba, E. prostrata*)
- Garlic (*Allium sativum*)
- Lavender (*Lavandula angustifolia*)
- Onion (*Allium cepa*)
- Rosemary (*Rosmarinus officinalis*)
- Saw palmetto (*Serenoa repens*)
- Soy (*Glycine max*)
- Tea (*Camellia sinensis*)

Head Lice

- Eucalyptus (*Eucalyptus globulus*)
- Lavender (*Lavandula angustifolia*)
- Neem (*Azadirachta indica*)
- Peppermint (*Mentha x piperita*)
- Tea tree (*Melaleuca alternifolia*)

Headache

- Butterbur (*Petasites hybridus*)
- Cayenne (*Capsicum annuum, C. frutescens*)
- Cramp bark (*Viburnum opulus*)
- Feverfew (*Tanacetum parthenium*)
- Lavender (*Lavandula angustifolia*)
- Willow (*Salix alba*)

Hemorrhoids

- Horse chestnut (*Aesculus hippocastanum*)
- Witch hazel (*Hamamelis virginiana*)

Hepatitis

See Liver Disease

High Blood Pressure (Hypertension)

- American ginseng (*Panax quinquefolius*)
- Cocoa (*Theobroma cacao*)
- Garlic (*Allium sativum*)
- Grape (*Vitis vinifera*)
- Maritime pine (*Pinus pinaster*)
- Pomegranate (*Punica granatum*)
- Turmeric (*Curcuma longa*)

High Blood Sugar (Hyperglycemia)

- Alfalfa (*Medicago sativa*)
- American ginseng (*Panax quinquefolius*)
- Amla (*Emblica officinalis, Phyllanthus emblica*)
- Ashwagandha (*Withania somnifera*)
- Asian ginseng (*Panax ginseng*)
- Astragalus (*Astragalus membranaceus*)
- Bilberry (*Vaccinium myrtillus*)
- Cinnamon (*Cinnamomum verum, C. aromaticum*)
- Eleuthero (*Eleutherococcus senticosus*)
- Fenugreek (*Trigonella foenum-graecum*)
- Gymnema (*Gymnema sylvestre*)
- Konjac (*Amorphophallus konjac, A. rivieri*)
- Oats (*Avena sativa*)

High Cholesterol (Hyperlipidemia)

- Alfalfa (*Medicago sativa*)
- Amla (*Emblica officinalis, Phyllanthus emblica*)
- Artichoke (*Cynara cardunculus, C. scolymus*)
- Astragalus (*Astragalus membranaceus*)
- Cocoa (*Theobroma cacao*)
- Fenugreek (*Trigonella foenum-graecum*)
- Flax (*Linum usitatissimum*)
- Garlic (*Allium sativum*)
- Goji-berry (*Lycium barbarum, L. chinense*)
- Oats (*Avena sativa*)
- Psyllium (*Plantago ovata, P. psyllium*)
- Rice bran (*Oryza sativa*)
- Soy (*Glycine max*)

Immune Support

- Ashwagandha (*Withania somnifera*)
- Asian ginseng (*Panax ginseng*)
- Cordyceps (*Cordyceps sinensis*)
- Licorice (*Glycyrrhiza glabra*)
- Rhodiola (*Rhodiola rosea*)
- Schisandra (*Schisandra chinensis*)
- Tulsi (*Ocimum tenuiflorum, O. sanctum*)

Indigestion and Upset Stomach

- Chamomile (*Matricaria recutita*)
- Fennel (*Foeniculum vulgare*)
- Ginger (*Zingiber officinale*)
- Peppermint (*Mentha x piperita*)
- Rosemary (*Rosmarinus officinalis*)

Infantile Colic

- Chamomile (*Matricaria recutita*)
- Lavender (*Lavandula angustifolia*)

Infectious Diseases

- Barberry (*Berberis vulgaris*)
- Lemon balm (*Melissa officinalis*)
- Reishi (*Ganoderma lucidum*)
- Tulsi (*Ocimum tenuiflorum, O. sanctum*)

Infertility (Female)

- Rhodiola (*Rhodiola rosea*)
- Vitex (*Vitex agnus-castus*)

Infertility (Male)

- Astragalus (*Astragalus membranaceus*)
- Eleuthero (*Eleutherococcus senticosus*)
- Goji-berry (*Lycium barbarum, L. chinense*)

Inflammatory Bowel Disease

- Boswellia (*Boswellia serrata*)
- Pineapple (*Ananas comosus*)

Inflammatory Skin Disorders

- Aloe (*Aloe vera*)
- Gotu kola (*Centella asiatica*)
- Licorice (*Glycyrrhiza glabra*)
- Oats (*Avena sativa*)
- Saint John's wort (*Hypericum perforatum*)
- Tea (*Camellia sinensis*)

Insect Bites and Stings

- Arnica (*Arnica montana*)
- Camphor (*Cinnamomum camphora*)
- Echinacea (*Echinacea purpurea*)
- Eucalyptus (*Eucalyptus globulus*)
- Sangre de grado (*Croton lechleri*)
- Tea tree (*Melaleuca alternifolia*)
- Witch hazel (*Hamamelis virginiana*)

Insect Repellant

- Camphor (*Cinnamomum camphora*)
- Cinnamon (*Cinnamomum verum, C. aromaticum*)
- Fennel (*Foeniculum vulgare*)
- Ginger (*Zingiber officinale*)
- Neem (*Azadirachta indica*)

Insomnia

- Ashwagandha (*Withania somnifera*)
- Chamomile (*Matricaria recutita*)
- Hops (*Humulus lupulus*)
- Kava (*Piper methysticum*)
- Lavender (*Lavandula angustifolia*)
- Lemon balm (*Melissa officinalis*)
- Passionflower (*Passiflora incarnata*)
- Valerian (*Valeriana officinalis*)

Irritable Bowel Syndrome

- Artichoke (*Cynara cardunculus, C. scolymus*)
- Peppermint (*Mentha x piperita*)

Liver Disease
- Milk thistle (*Silybum marianum*)
- Schisandra (*Schisandra chinensis*)

Liver Support
- Artichoke (*Cynara cardunculus,
  C. scolymus*)
- Milk thistle (*Silybum marianum*)

Loss of Appetite
- Dandelion (*Taraxucum officinale*)
- Fenugreek (*Trigonella foenum-graecum*)

Low Energy
- American ginseng (*Panax quinquefolius*)
- Asian ginseng (*Panax ginseng*)
- Coffee (*Coffea arabica*)
- Guarana (*Paullinia cupana*)
- Maca (*Lepidium meyenii*)
- Mate (*Ilex paraguariensis*)
- Rhodiola (*Rhodiola rosea*)
- Tea (*Camellia sinensis*)

Macular Degeneration
    See Age-Related Eye Disease

Menopausal Symptoms
- Black cohosh (*Actaea racemosa,
  Cimicifuga racemosa*)
- Dong quai (*Angelica sinensis*)
- Flax (*Linum usitatissimum*)
- Kava (*Piper methysticum*)
- Kudzu (*Pueraria lobata*)
- Red clover (*Trifolium pratense*)
- Soy (*Glycine max*)
- Saint John's wort (*Hypericum
  perforatum*)

Menstrual Symptoms and PMS
- Cramp bark (*Viburnum opulus*)
- Ginkgo (*Ginkgo biloba*)
- Maritime pine (*Pinus pinaster*)
- Saint John's wort (*Hypericum
  perforatum*)
- Vitex (*Vitex agnus-castus*)

Migraine Headache
    See Headache

Minor Wounds
- Aloe (*Aloe vera*)
- Amla (*Emblica officinalis, Phyllanthus
  emblica*)
- Barberry (*Berberis vulgaris*)
- Calendula (*Calendula officinalis*)
- Chamomile (*Matricaria recutita*)
- Echinacea (*Echinacea purpurea*)
- Eucalyptus (*Eucalyptus globulus*)
- Garlic (*Allium sativum*)
- Gotu kola (*Centella asiatica*)
- Horsetail (*Equisetum arvense*)
- Lavender (*Lavandula angustifolia*)
- Marshmallow (*Althaea officinalis*)
- Sangre de grado (*Croton lechleri*)
- Saint John's wort (*Hypericum
  perforatum*)
- Tea tree (*Melaleuca alternifolia*)
- Yarrow (*Achillea millefolium*)

Muscle and Joint Pain
- Arnica (*Arnica montana*)
- Camphor (*Cinnamomum camphora*)
- Cayenne (*Capsicum annuum,
  C. frutescens*)
- Comfrey (*Symphytum officinale*)
- Eucalyptus (*Eucalyptus globulus*)
- Ginger (*Zingiber officinale*)
- Pineapple (*Ananas comosus*)
- Rosemary (*Rosmarinus officinalis*)
- Yarrow (*Achillea millefolium*)

Nausea and Vomiting
- Cinnamon (*Cinnamomum verum,
  C. aromaticum*)
- Ginger (*Zingiber officinale*)
- Lavender (*Lavandula angustifolia*)
- Rooibos (*Aspalathus linearis*)

Obesity
    See Weight Loss

Oily Hair and Scalp
- Juniper (*Juniperus communis*)
- Willow (*Salix alba*)
- Witch hazel (*Hamamelis virginiana*)

Oily Skin
- Calendula (*Calendula officinalis*)
- Juniper (*Juniperus communis*)
- Tea tree (*Melaleuca alternifolia*)
- Witch hazel (*Hamamelis virginiana*)

Oral Care
- Clove (*Syzygium aromaticum*)
- Fennel (*Foeniculum vulgare*)
- Neem (*Azadirachta indica*)
- Peppermint (*Mentha x piperita*)
- Tea (*Camellia sinensis*)
- Tea tree (*Melaleuca alternifolia*)

Oral Pain
- Clove (*Syzygium aromaticum*)
- Slippery elm (*Ulmus rubra*)
- Tea tree (*Melaleuca alternifolia*)

Osteoporosis
- Evening primrose (*Oenothera biennis*)
- Red clover (*Trifolium pratense*)
- Soy (*Glycine max*)
- Tea (*Camellia sinensis*)

Pregnancy-Related Discomfort
- Cayenne (*Capsicum annuum, C. frutescens*)
- Ginger (*Zingiber officinale*)
- Maritime pine (*Pinus pinaster*)
- Peppermint (*Mentha x piperita*)
- Psyllium (*Plantago ovata, P. psyllium*)
- Witch hazel (*Hamamelis virginiana*)

Psoriasis
See Inflammatory Skin Disorders

Rheumatoid Arthritis
- Borage (*Borago officinalis*)
- Cayenne (*Capsicum annuum, C. frutescens*)
- Feverfew (*Tanacetum parthenium*)
- Ginger (*Zingiber officinale*)
- Grape (*Vitis vinifera*)

Ringworm
- Camphor (*Cinnamomum camphora*)
- Clove (*Syzygium aromaticum*)
- Echinacea (*Echinacea purpurea*)
- Garlic (*Allium sativum*)
- Lavender (*Lavandula angustifolia*)
- Tea tree (*Melaleuca alternifolia*)

Rosacea
See Inflammatory Skin Disorders

Scars
- Cocoa (*Theobroma cacao*)
- Gotu kola (*Centella asiatica*)
- Onion (*Allium cepa*)

Sexual Dysfunction (Female)
- Ashwagandha (*Withania somnifera*)
- Yohimbe (*Pausinystalia yohimbe*)

Sexual Dysfunction (Male)
- Asian ginseng (*Panax ginseng*)
- Ginkgo (*Ginkgo biloba*)
- Goji-berry (*Lycium barbarum, L. chinense*)
- Kava (*Piper methysticum*)
- Maca (*Lepidium meyenii*)
- Maritime pine (*Pinus pinaster*)
- Schisandra (*Schisandra chinensis*)
- Yohimbe (*Pausinystalia yohimbe*)

Sexually Transmitted Diseases
See Infectious Diseases

Sore Throat
See Cough and Sore Throat

Sprains and Strains
- Arnica (*Arnica montana*)
- Comfrey (*Symphytum officinale*)
- Pineapple (*Ananas comosus*)

Stimulant
- Coffee (*Coffea arabica*)
- Guarana (*Paullinia cupana*)
- Mate (*Ilex paraguariensis*)
- Tea (*Camellia sinensis*)

Stress
- American ginseng (*Panax quinquefolius*)
- Amla (*Emblica officinalis, Phyllanthus emblica*)
- Ashwagandha (*Withania somnifera*)
- Asian ginseng (*Panax ginseng*)
- Astragalus (*Astragalus membranaceus*)
- Cordyceps (*Cordyceps sinensis*)
- Eleuthero (*Eleutherococcus senticosus*)
- Goji-berry (*Lycium barbarum, L. chinense*)
- Licorice (*Glycyrrhiza glabra*)
- Maca (*Lepidium meyenii*)
- Reishi (*Ganoderma lucidum*)
- Rhodiola (*Rhodiola rosea*)
- Schisandra (*Schisandra chinensis*)
- Tulsi (*Ocimum tenuiflorum, O. sanctum*)
- Saint John's wort (*Hypericum perforatum*)

Stretch Marks
See Scars

Sunburn
See Burns

Sun Protection
- Coffee (*Coffea arabica*)
- Grape (*Vitis vinifera*)
- Maca (*Lepidium meyenii*)
- Maritime pine (*Pinus pinaster*)
- Olive (*Olea europaea*)
- Rose (*Rosa damascena, R. canina, R. spp.*)
- Tea (*Camellia sinensis*)

Teething
- Chamomile (*Matricaria recutita*)
- Slippery elm (*Ulmus rubra*)

Ulcerative Colitis
See Inflammatory Bowel Disease

Ulcers (Peptic)
- Aloe (*Aloe vera*)
- Cat's claw (*Uncaria guianensis, U. tomentosa*)
- Gotu kola (*Centella asiatica*)
- Licorice (*Glycyrrhiza glabra*)
- Neem (*Azadirachta indica*)

Urinary Tract Infection
- Coleus (*Coleus forskohlii, Plectranthus barbatus*)
- Dandelion (*Taraxucum officinale*)
- Grapefruit (*Citrus paradisi*)
- Juniper (*Juniperus communis*)

Varicose Veins
- Bilberry (*Vaccinium myrtillus*)
- Butcher's broom (*Ruscus aculeatus*)
- Gotu kola (*Centella asiatica*)
- Grape (*Vitis vinifera*)
- Horse chestnut (*Aesculus hippocastanum*)
- Maritime pine (*Pinus pinaster*)

Viral Infection
- Aloe (*Aloe vera*)
- Barberry (*Berberis vulgaris*)
- Cat's claw (*Uncaria guianensis, U. tomentosa*)
- Echinacea (*Echinacea purpurea*)
- Lemon balm (*Melissa officinalis*)
- Licorice (*Glycyrrhiza glabra*)
- Peppermint (*Mentha x piperita*)
- Tea (*Camellia sinensis*)

Vision Support
- Bilberry (*Vaccinium myrtillus*)
- Grape (*Vitis vinifera*)
- Maritime pine (*Pinus pinaster*)

Warts
- Garlic (*Allium sativum*)
- Tea (*Camellia sinensis*)

Weight Loss
- Cayenne (*Capsicum annuum, C. frutescens*)
- Clove (*Syzygium aromaticum*)
- Coffee (*Coffea arabica*)
- Coleus (*Coleus forskohlii, Plectranthus barbatus*)
- Eucalyptus (*Eucalyptus globulus*)
- Garcinia (*Garcinia cambogia, G. gummi-gutta*)
- Ginger (*Zingiber officinale*)
- Grapefruit (*Citrus paradisi*)
- Guarana (*Paullinia cupana*)
- Gymnema (*Gymnema sylvestre*)
- Konjac (*Amorphophallus konjac, A. rivieri*)
- Maritime pine (*Pinus pinaster*)
- Mate (*Ilex paraguariensis*)
- Pomegranate (*Punica granatum*)
- Psyllium (*Plantago ovata, P. psyllium*)
- Soy (*Glycine max*)
- Tea (*Camellia sinensis*)
- Turmeric (*Curcuma longa*)

Yeast Infection (Candidiasis)
- Echinacea (*Echinacea purpurea*)
- Goldenseal (*Hydrastis canadensis*)
- Tea tree (*Melaleuca alternifolia*)

Popular Herbs A–Z

Name	Medicinal Parts	Key Uses	Available Forms	Safety Issues and Advice
Alfalfa (*Medicago sativa*)	leaf, seed	bloating and water retention, gas and flatulence, diabetes, hyperglycemia, hyperlipidemia	bulk, capsules, juice, powder, tablets, tea	Anticoagulant/antiplatelet, cholesterol-lowering, hypoglycemic, immunomodulating potential (see Chapter 17).
Aloe (*Aloe vera*)	leaf	Internal: constipation, diabetes, hyperglycemia, ulcers; External: bacterial, fungal, or viral infection; burns; cold sores; inflammatory skin disorders, minor wounds	bulk, capsules, cream, gel, lotion, powder, juice, tablets	Aloe gel is used internally and topically (don't apply to deep wounds). Latex, a sap from the outer rind, is used internally. Aloe gel has hypoglycemic potential when taken internally. Don't take aloe latex if you have chronic gastrointestinal or kidney problems, are pregnant or nursing, or take heart medications; don't combine with other laxatives.
American ginseng (*Panax quinquefolius*)	root	athletic performance, colds and flu, hyperglycemia, hypertension, low energy, stress	capsules, tablets, tincture	Hypoglycemic, estrogenic potential (see Chapter 17). Buy organically grown American ginseng—it's threatened in the wild. If using long term, stop taking for two weeks every three months.
Amla (*Emblica officinalis, Phyllanthus emblica*); also known as amalaki or Indian gooseberry	fruit, leaf, bark	Internal: diabetes, hyperglycemia, hyperlipidemia, stress; External: hair care, hair color, minor wounds	capsules, juice, tablets, cream, herbal oil, ointment, powder	Amla contains tannins, which might exacerbate a case of diarrhea.
Andrographis (*Andrographis paniculata*)	leaf, rhizome	colds and flu	capsules, tablets	Anticoagulant/antiplatelet, hypotensive, immunomodulating potential (see Chapter 17).
Arnica (*Arnica montana*)	flower	Internal (homeopathic): muscle and joint pain; External (herbal and homeopathic): bruises, insect bites and stings, muscle and joint pain, sprains and strains	homeopathic pills/pellets, cream, gel, ointment, tincture	Anticoagulant/antiplatelet potential; allergenic potential as a member of the *Asteraceae/ Compositae* family (see Chapter 17). Don't take herbal arnica internally and don't apply to broken skin.
Artichoke (*Cynara cardunculus, C. scolymus*)	leaf, stem, root	acid indigestion (dyspepsia), gas and flatulence, hyperlipidemia, irritable bowel syndrome, liver support	capsules, tablets, tincture	*Asteraceae/Compositae* family (see Chapter 17). If you have gallstones, talk to your doctor before using.
Ashwagandha (*Withania somnifera*)	root, fruit	anxiety, arthritis, autoimmune disorders, diabetes/hyperglycemia, female sexual dysfunction, immune support, insomnia, stress	capsules, liquid extract, tablets, tea	Hypoglycemic, immunomodulating, sedative potential (see Chapter 17). Avoid if you're pregnant, are taking antianxiety medications, or have peptic ulcers.

Name	Medicinal Parts	Key Uses	Available Forms	Safety Issues and Advice
Asian ginseng (*Panax ginseng*)	root	altitude sickness, athletic performance, autoimmune disorders, cognitive function and memory, diabetes, hyperglycemia, immune support, low energy, male sexual dysfunction, stress	bulk, capsules, liquid extract, powder, tablets, tea, tincture	Anticoagulant/antiplatelet, cardioactive, estrogenic, hypoglycemic, immunomodulating, stimulant potential (see Chapter 17). Every three months, stop taking for two weeks.
Astragalus (*Astragalus membranaceus*)	root	atopic dermatitis, autoimmune disorders, cancer, diabetes, hyperglycemia, hepatitis (chronic), hyperlipidemia, male infertility, stress	bulk, capsules, liquid extract, powder, tablets, tea, tincture	Immunomodulating potential (see Chapter 17).
Barberry (*Berberis vulgaris*)	fruit, bark, root, root bark	Internal: diarrhea, infectious disease; External: bacterial, fungal, viral infection; minor wounds	capsules, liquid extract, tincture	Antimicrobial action strongest when used externally. Avoid oral preparations if you're pregnant.
Bilberry (*Vaccinium myrtillus*)	fruit, leaf	age-related eye disease, autoimmune disorders, hyperglycemia, varicose veins, vision support	capsules, liquid extract, tablets, tea	Hypoglycemic potential (see Chapter 17). Don't combine with antiplatelet/anticoagulant drugs. Standardized products typically contain 25 percent anthocyanins/anthocyanocides.
Black cohosh (*Actaea racemosa*, *Cimicifuga racemosa*)	rhizome, root	menopausal symptoms	capsules, liquid extract, tablets, tea, cream	Estrogenic, hepatotoxic potential (see Chapter 17). Can cause stomach upset (take with food). Black cohosh is threatened; buy organically grown products.
Borage (*Borago officinalis*)	seed	Internal: rheumatoid arthritis; External: dry skin	capsules, cream, lotion	Anticoagulant/antiplatelet, hepatotoxic potential (see Chapter 17). Pregnant women should avoid.
Boswellia (*Boswellia serrata*); also known as Indian frankincense	trunk (resin)	Internal: age-related eye disease, arthritis, asthma, inflammatory bowel disease; External: anxiety, depression	capsules, tablets, essential oil, herbal oil, cream	Can cause gastrointestinal problems and skin reactions.
Bromelain: See Pineapple				
Butcher's broom (*Ruscus aculeatus*)	rhizome, root	varicose veins	capsules, tablets	Can cause stomach upset. Works best when combined with vitamin C.
Butterbur (*Petasites hybridus*)	leaf, rhizome, root	allergies, headache	capsules	Hepatotoxic potential; *Asteraceae/Compositae* family (see Chapter 17). Can cause stomach upset.
Calendula (*Calendula officinalis*)	flower	acne, burns, canker sores, cuts and scrapes, diaper rash, minor wounds, oily skin	bulk, cream, essential oil, herbal oil, homeopathic preparations, liquid extract, lotion	Sedative potential; *Asteraceae/Compositae* family (see Chapter 17). Pregnant women should avoid oral preparations.

Name	Medicinal Parts	Key Uses	Available Forms	Safety Issues and Advice
Camphor (*Cinnamomum camphora*)	bark, wood	arthritis, athlete's foot, burns, cough, deodorant, insect bites and stings, fungal infection, insect repellant, muscle and joint pain	essential oil, herbal oil, ointment	Don't take internally, and don't use on children. Dilute essential oil before using. Don't apply to broken skin.
Cat's claw (*Uncaria guianensis, U. tomentosa*)	root, bark	arthritis, bacterial and viral infection, ulcers	capsules, liquid extract	Hypotensive, immunomodulating potential (see Chapter 17). Avoid if you're pregnant.
Cayenne (*Capsicum annuum, C. frutescens*)	fruit	Internal: weight loss; External: arthritis, headache, muscle and joint pain, pregnancy-related discomfort, rheumatoid arthritis	capsules, liquid extract, cream, herbal oil, ointment	Anticoagulant/antiplatelet potential; contains salicylates (see Chapter 17). Don't use on young children and don't apply to broken skin (avoid your eyes). Pregnant or breastfeeding women shouldn't take orally.
Chamomile (*Matricaria recutita*)	flower	Internal: acid indigestion (dyspepsia), anxiety, digestion support, indigestion and upset stomach, infantile colic, insomnia; External: minor wounds, teething	bulk, capsules, essential oil, herbal oil, liquid extract, lotion, tea, cream	Anticoagulant/antiplatelet, antiestrogenic, sedative potential; *Asteraceae/Compositae* family (see Chapter 17). Avoid internal preparations if you're taking antianxiety drugs.
Cinnamon (*Cinnamomum verum, C. aromaticum*)	bark	Internal: digestion support, hyperglycemia, nausea and vomiting; External: insect repellant	bulk, capsules, powder, tablets, tea, essential oil	Hepatotoxic, hypoglycemic potential; contains salicylates (see Chapter 17). Dilute essential oil before using, and don't take internally.
Clove (*Syzygium aromaticum*)	dried flower bud, leaf, stem	Internal: weight loss; External: bacterial, fungal, viral infection; canker sores; cold sores; oral care; oral pain; ringworm	bulk, essential oil, powder, tea	Contains salicylates (see Chapter 17). Large doses can be toxic; topical application can cause skin reactions. Don't apply to broken skin and don't use on young children.
Cocoa (*Theobroma cacao*)	seed	Internal: age-related cognitive decline, hyperlipidemia, hypertension; External: dry skin, scars	capsules, liquid extract, powdered herb, cream (cocoa butter)	Stimulant (see Chapter 17). Cocoa butter can cause skin reactions.
Coffee (*Coffea arabica*)	bean	Internal: asthma, athletic performance, headache, low energy, weight loss; External: aging skin; sun protection	bulk, liquid extract	Stimulant (see Chapter 17).
Coleus (*Coleus forskohlii, Plectranthus barbatus*); also known as forskolin	root	urinary tract infection, weight loss	capsules, liquid extract	Antiplatelet/anticoagulant, cardioactive potential (see Chapter 17).
Comfrey (*Symphytum officinale*)	leaf, rhizome, root	bruises, muscle and joint pain, sprains and strains	bulk, cream, ointment	Hepatotoxic potential (see Chapter 17). Don't take internally. Avoid if pregnant or nursing.
Cordyceps (*Cordyceps sinensis*)	mushroom	asthma, athletic performance, cancer, chronic obstructive pulmonary disease (COPD), immune support, stress	capsules, liquid extract, tablets	Immunomodulating (see Chapter 17).

Name	Medicinal Parts	Key Uses	Available Forms	Safety Issues and Advice
Cramp bark (*Viburnum opulus*)	bark, root bark	back pain, headache, menstrual symptoms and PMS	capsules, tablets, tincture	No known interactions or side effects.
Dandelion (*Taraxucum officinale*)	leaf, root	bloating and water retention, loss of appetite, urinary tract infection	capsules, liquid extract, tea, tincture	*Asteraceae/Compositae* family (see Chapter 17).
Danshen (*Salvia miltiorrhiza*)	root	addictions and alcoholism, cardiovascular disease	capsules, tablets	Anticoagulant/antiplatelet, cardioactive potential (see Chapter 17). Can cause stomach upset.
Devil's claw (*Harpagphytum procumbens*)	root	arthritis, back pain	capsules, liquid extract	Cardioactive (see Chapter 17). Avoid if you're prone to acid reflux or are taking antidyspepsia drugs.
Dong quai (*Angelica sinensis*)	root	menopausal symptoms	capsules, liquid extract, powder, tea, tincture	Anticoagulant/antiplatelet, estrogenic potential (see Chapter 17).
Echinacea (*Echinacea purpurea*)	aerial parts, root	Internal: allergies, athlete's foot, colds and flu, ringworm, fungal and viral infection; External: insect bites and stings, minor wounds, poisonous plants, viral infection	bulk, capsules, liquid extract, tincture	Immunomodulating. *Asteraceae/Compositae* family (see Chapter 17). Preparations made from the root seem to have the best effect. Buy only organically grown echinacea; it's threatened in the wild.
Eclipta (*Eclipta alba*, *E. prostrata*)	leaf	hair care, hair color, hair loss	juice, herbal oil, powder	*Asteraceae/Compositae* family (see Chapter 17).
Elderberry (*Sambucus nigra*)	fruit	colds and flu	capsules, liquid extract	Immunomodulating (see Chapter 17).
Eleuthero (*Eleutherococcus senticosus*), also known as Siberian ginseng	root	athletic performance, hyperglycemia, male infertility, stress, viral infection	capsules, liquid extract, tea, tincture	Anticoagulant/antiplatelet, hypoglycemic, immunomodulating, sedative potential (see Chapter 17). Eleuthero is often recommended for people who find Asian ginseng too stimulating.
Eucalyptus (*Eucalyptus globulus*)	leaf, oil (leaf, branches)	Internal: asthma, colds and flu, weight loss; External: cough and sore throat, cuts and scrapes, head lice, insect bites and stings, minor wounds, muscle and joint pain, poisonous plants	bulk, capsules, liquid extract, tea, essential oil, herbal oil, lotion, ointment	Hypoglycemic potential (see Chapter 17). Undiluted eucalyptus oil is extremely toxic. If you want an oral remedy, use only products labeled for internal use (they're made with leaf extracts or minute amounts of oil)
Evening primrose (*Oenothera biennis*)	seed	Internal: breast pain (mastaglia), cancer, osteoporosis; External: aging skin, dry skin	capsules, herbal oil, cream, lotion	Anticoagulant/antiplatelet potential (see Chapter 17). Don't use orally if you're pregnant.
Fennel (*Foeniculum vulgare*)	seed	Internal: digestion support, gas and flatulence, indigestion and upset stomach; External: insect repellant, oral care	bulk, capsules, essential oil, powder, tea, tincture	Estrogenic potential (see Chapter 17). Don't use oil undiluted.
Fenugreek (*Trigonella foenum-graecum*)	seed	constipation, diabetes, hyperglycemia, hyperlipidemia, loss of appetite	capsules, ground seeds, tea	Anticoagulant/antiplatelet, hypoglycemic potential; contains salicylates (see Chapter 17). Excessive doses can cause diarrhea.

Name	Medicinal Parts	Key Uses	Available Forms	Safety Issues and Advice
Feverfew (*Tanacetum parthenium*)	leaf	autoimmune disorders, headache, rheumatoid arthritis	bulk, capsules, liquid extract, tablets	Anticoagulant/antiplatelet potential; *Asteraceae/ Compositae* family (see Chapter 17). Avoid during pregnancy.
Flax (*Linum usitatissimum*)	seed	Internal: ADHD, age-related eye disease, autoimmune disorders, constipation, hyperlipidemia, menopausal symptoms; External: dry hair and skin	bulk, capsules, herbal oil, powder, cream, lotion	Hypoglycemic, cholesterol-lowering, estrogenic potential (see Chapter 17). Excessive doses can cause bloating and diarrhea. Store in the refrigerator.
Forskolin: See Coleus				
Garcinia (*Garcinia cambogia, G. gummi-gutta*)	fruit, rind	weight loss	capsules, tablets	Can cause nausea and headaches.
Garlic (*Allium sativum*)	bulb (root)	Internal: age-related cognitive decline, Alzheimer's disease and dementia, colds and flu, digestion support, disease prevention, hyperlipidemia, hypertension; External: athlete's foot; bacterial, fungal, and viral infection; cold sores; cuts and scrapes; ear infection; hair loss; minor wounds; ringworm; warts	bulk, capsules, herbal oil, liquid extract, powder, tablets, tincture	Anticoagulant/antiplatelet, cholesterol-lowering, hypotensive potential (see Chapter 17). Avoid if you have chronic or inflammatory gastrointestinal problems. Garlic can interfere with several prescription medicines; talk with your doctor if you're on long-term drug therapy. If you're using fresh garlic, eat at least four cloves a day (crush to release the active constituents). Standardized products typically contain at least 1 percent allicin (or at least 4 mgs per dose) and 1 percent alliin.
Ginger (*Zingiber officinale*)	rhizome	Internal: arthritis, autoimmune disorders, back pain, cancer, colds and flu, cough and sore throat, foodborne illness (food poisoning), muscle and joint pain, indigestion and upset stomach, nausea and vomiting, pregnancy-related discomfort, rheumatoid arthritis, weight loss; External: back pain, insect repellant, muscle and joint pain	bulk, capsules, essential oil, liquid extract, powder, syrup, tea, tincture, essential oil	Anticoagulant/antiplatelet, hypoglycemic potential; contains salicylates (see Chapter 17). Can cause stomach upset and diarrhea (don't take more than 5 grams a day).
Ginkgo (*Ginkgo biloba*)	leaf, seed	ADHD, addictions and alcoholism, age-related cognitive decline, age-related eye disease, altitude sickness, Alzheimer's disease and dementia, asthma, male sexual dysfunction, menstrual symptoms and PMS	capsules, liquid extract, tablets, tea, tincture	Anticoagulant/antiplatelet (see Chapter 17). Don't take if you're pregnant or taking anticonvulsant, antidiabetes, or antidepressant drugs or herbs. Products are typically standardized to contain 24 to 25 percent glycosides and 6 percent terpenoids. It may take up to eight weeks to see results.
Goji-berry (*Lycium barbarum, L. chinense*); also known as lycium or Chinese wolfberry	dried berry, root bark	hyperlipidemia, male infertility, male sexual dysfunction, stress	bulk, capsules, juice, liquid extract, tablets, tea	Root bark has hypoglycemic and hypotensive potential (see Chapter 17). Avoid if you're sensitive to other plants in the nightshade family (including tomatoes and eggplant). Use caution if taking with anticoagulants. Buy berries grown organically in the United States; some imported Chinese berries are contaminated with pesticides.

Name	Medicinal Parts	Key Uses	Available Forms	Safety Issues and Advice
Goldenseal (*Hydrastis canadensis*)	rhizome, root	Internal: bacterial infection, ear infection; External: yeast infection (candidiasis), ear infection	capsules, liquid extract, tablets, tea, tincture	Goldenseal's antimicrobial effects seem strongest when it's used topically. Pregnant women shouldn't use goldenseal. Goldenseal is threatened; buy organically grown products.
Gotu kola (*Centella asiatica*)	aerial parts	Internal: ulcers, varicose veins; External: aging skin, bacterial infection, cuts and scrapes, inflammatory skin disorders, minor wounds, scars	capsules, liquid extract, powder, tea, tincture, cream, lotion	Hepatotoxic, sedative potential (see Chapter 17).
Grape (*Vitis vinifera*)	leaf, seed, skin (fruit)	Internal: age-related cognitive decline, age-related eye disease, Alzheimer's disease and dementia, autoimmune disorders, cancer, cardiovascular disease, chronic venous insufficiency, disease prevention, hypertension, rheumatoid arthritis, sun protection, varicose veins, vision support; External: aging skin, sun protection	capsules, juice, liquid extract, tablets, wine, cream, herbal oil, lotion	Grape skins contain salicylates (see Chapter 17). Standardized grape seed extracts typically contain 95 percent proanthocyanidins.
Grapefruit (*Citrus paradisi*)	fruit, juice, peel, seed	asthma, urinary tract infection (seed), weight loss	bulk, capsules, essential oil (peel), juice, liquid extract (seed), powder (pectin), tablets	Contains salicylates (see Chapter 17). Can cause serious interactions with several drugs; talk with your doctor before using.
Guarana (*Paullinia cupana*)	seed	asthma, athletic performance, low energy, weight loss	capsules, drink, liquid extract, powder, tablets	Stimulant (see Chapter 17); guarana contains roughly three times the caffeine of coffee.
Guggul (*Commiphora wightii, C. mukul*)	trunk (resin)	acne, arthritis	capsules, tablets	Anticoagulant/antiplatelet, cholesterol-lowering, estrogenic potential (see Chapter 17). Gum guggul can cause reactions; look for extracts called *guggulipid*, which are more effective and aren't associated with side effects. Avoid during pregnancy. Check with your doctor before combining with prescription drugs.
Gymnema (*Gymnema sylvestre*)	leaf	Diabetes, hyperglycemia, weight loss	capsules, liquid extract, powder, tablets, tea, tincture	Hypogylcemic potential (see Chapter 17).
Hawthorn (*Crataegus monogyna, C. oxyacantha*)	flower, fruit, leaf	cardiovascular disease	bulk, capsules, liquid extract, tablets, tea, tincture	Cardioactive, cholesterol-lowering, hypotensive potential (see Chapter 17). Don't use if you're pregnant. Products are standardized to contain roughly 2 percent flavonoids and 19 percent oligomeric procyanidins (OPCs). You might have to use hawthorn for several weeks before you notice a benefit.

Name	Medicinal Parts	Key Uses	Available Forms	Safety Issues and Advice
Hops (*Humulus lupulus*)	flower	allergies, anxiety, atopic dermatitis, digestion support, insomnia	capsule, liquid extract, tea, tincture	Sedative (see Chapter 17).
Horse chestnut (*Aesculus hippocastanum*)	seed	Internal: chronic venous insufficiency, hemorrhoids, varicose veins; External: hemorrhoids, varicose veins	capsules, tablets, cream, gel, lotion	Anticoagulant/antiplatelet, hypoglycemic potential (see Chapter 17).
Horsetail (*Equisetum arvense*)	aerial parts	Cuts and scrapes, hair care, minor wounds	liquid extract, tea	Don't use if you're pregnant. Don't use crude (unprocessed) herbal preparations internally (they can be toxic).
Jojoba (*Simmondsia chinensis*)	seed	dry hair and skin	cream, lotion, oil	Don't take jojoba oil internally.
Juniper (*Juniperus communis*)	berry	Internal: bloating and water retention, diarrhea, foodborne illness (food poisoning), urinary tract infection; External: acne, dandruff, deodorant, oily hair and skin	bulk, capsules, liquid extract, tea, tincture, essential oil	Juniper can cause skin irritation. Do not apply essential oil undiluted and don't take internally. Pregnant women should avoid all oral juniper preparations.
Kava (*Piper methysticum*)	root	anxiety, insomnia, male sexual dysfunction, menopausal symptoms	capsules, liquid extract, powder, tea, tincture	Hepatotoxic, sedative (see Chapter 17). Kava is controversial (the FDA has issued a warning about kava, and it's been banned in Canada and Germany). Pregnant women shouldn't take kava. Don't combine with antidepressants or antianxiety drugs. Don't exceed recommended doses or use long term. Products are standardized to contain at least 15 percent kavalactones (some contain as much as 70 percent). Kava is threatened in the wild; buy organically grown.
Konjac (*Amorphophallus konjac, A. rivieri*)	root	constipation, diabetes, hyperglycemia, weight loss	capsules	Hypoglycemic, cholesterol-lowering potential (see Chapter 17).
Kudzu (*Pueraria lobata*)	root, flower, leaf	addictions and alcoholism, menopausal symptoms	capsules, powder, tablets, tincture	Anticoagulant/antiplatelet, hypoglycemic, estrogenic potential (see Chapter 17).
Lavender (*Lavandula angustifolia*)	flower	Internal: acid indigestion (dyspepsia), anxiety, depression, digestion support, gas and flatulence, insomnia, nausea and vomiting; External: anxiety, athlete's foot, back pain, burns, ear infection, diaper rash, fungal infection, hair loss, headache, head lice, infantile colic, insomnia, minor wounds, ringworm	bulk, capsules, liquid extract, tea, essential oil, cream, lotion	Don't use lavender essential oil internally.

Name	Medicinal Parts	Key Uses	Available Forms	Safety Issues and Advice
Lemon balm (*Melissa officinalis*); also known as Melissa	leaf	Internal: acid indigestion (dyspepsia), Alzheimer's disease and dementia, anxiety, depression, insomnia; External: cold sores, infectious diseases, viral infection	bulk, capsules, liquid extract, powder, tablets, tincture, essential oil, salve, tea	Sedative (see Chapter 17). Don't take the essential oil internally.
Licorice (*Glycyrrhiza glabra*)	root	Internal: acid indigestion (dyspepsia), allergies, autoimmune disease (secondary infection), colds and flu, immune support, stress, ulcers; External: cold sores, dandruff, inflammatory skin disorders, viral infection	bulk, capsules, liquid extract, lozenges, tablets, tea, tincture	Anticoagulant/antiplatelet, hypertensive potential; contains salicylates (see Chapter 17). The chemical glycyrrhizin can raise your blood pressure and cause toxicity—deglycyrrhizinated licorice (DGL) is considered safer but may be less effective against allergies and systemic infection. Don't use internally if you're pregnant or have heart or kidney problems.
Maca (*Lepidium meyenii*)	root	Internal: low energy, male sexual dysfunction, stress; External: sun protection	capsules, liquid extract, powder, tablets, tincture	Maca has no known interactions or side effects.
Maritime pine (*Pinus pinaster*)	bark	ADHD, age-related eye disease, aging skin, asthma, athletic performance, chronic venous insufficiency, hypertension, male sexual dysfunction, menstrual symptoms and PMS, pregnancy-related discomfort, sun protection, varicose veins, vision support, weight loss	capsules, tablets	Immunomodulating (see Chapter 17).
Marshmallow (*Althaea officinalis*)	leaf, root	Internal: cough and sore throat, diarrhea; External: burns, cuts and scrapes, hair care, minor wounds	capsules, liquid extract, powder, tablet, tea	Hypoglycemic potential (see Chapter 17). Don't apply to open or deep wounds.
Mate (*Ilex paraguariensis*)	leaf, leaf stem	low energy, weight loss	bulk, capsules, tablets, tea	Stimulant (see Chapter 17).
Milk thistle (*Silybum marianum*)	aerial parts, seed	diabetes, hyperglycemia, liver disease, liver support	capsules, liquid extract, powder, tablets, tincture	*Asteraceae/Compositae* family (see Chapter 17). Can cause GI upset. Extracts are typically standardized for 70 to 80 percent silymarin.
Neem (*Azadirachta indica*)	bark, leaf, seed	Internal: ulcers; External: head lice, insect repellant, oral care	capsules, liquid extract, powder, tablets, cream, herbal oil, lotion, mouthwash, salve, shampoo, spray (insect repellant), toothpaste	Hypoglycemic, immunomodulating potential (see Chapter 17). Pregnant women and women trying to conceive shouldn't take neem internally (it's used as a form of birth control in India). Don't give oral neem to children.
Nettle (*Urtica dioica*)	aerial parts, root	Internal: allergies, arthritis, bloating and water retention, benign prostatic hyperplasia (BPH); External: arthritis, hair care	bulk, capsules, liquid extract, powder, tablets, tea, tincture, cream, lotion, shampoo	Hypoglycemic, hypotensive potential (see Chapter 17).

Name	Medicinal Parts	Key Uses	Available Forms	Safety Issues and Advice
Oats (*Avena sativa*)	bran, seed	Internal: digestion support, disease prevention, hyperglycemia, hyperlipidemia; External: atopic dermatitis, inflammatory skin disorders	bulk, liquid extract, tablets, cream, lotion, powder, soap	Cholesterol-lowering potential (see Chapter 17).
Olive (*Olea europaea*)	fruit	Internal: disease prevention, constipation, hyperlipidemia, hypertension; External: dry hair and skin, sun protection	oil, lotion, hair care products	Hypoglycemic, hypotensive potential (see Chapter 17).
Onion (*Allium cepa*)	bulb	Internal: cardiovascular disease; External: hair loss, scars	bulk, gel, juice, herbal oil, powder	Antiplatelet/anticoagulant, hypoglycemic potential (see Chapter 17).
Passionflower (*Passiflora incarnata*)	aerial parts	addictions and alcoholism, anxiety, insomnia	bulk, capsules, liquid extract, powder, tea, tincture	Sedative (see Chapter 17). Pregnant women should avoid passionflower.
Peppermint (*Mentha x piperita*)	aerial parts	Internal: acid indigestion (dyspepsia), digestion support, gas and flatulence, indigestion and upset stomach, irritable bowel syndrome, pregnancy-related discomfort, viral infection; External: colds and flu, oral care, dandruff, headache, head lice	bulk, capsules, powder, tea, essential oil, hair care products, lotion, oral care products	Contains salicylates (see Chapter 17). Can cause digestive upset; using enteric-coated capsules can help (take them between meals). Topical peppermint can cause irritation; always dilute essential oil before using (don't take internally).
Pineapple (*Ananas comosus*)	stem	Internal: acid indigestion (dyspepsia), arthritis, digestion support, inflammatory bowel disease, muscle and joint pain, sprains and strains; External: aging skin	capsules, tablets, commercial skin care products	Anticoagulant/antiplatelet potential (see Chapter 17). The beneficial ingredient in pineapple is the enzyme bromelain. If you're using it to treat a digestive complaint, take it with food; if you're using it for something else, take it on an empty stomach.
Pomegranate (*Punica granatum*)	leaf, fruit (juice, rind, seed), bark (root, stem), root	Internal: cardiovascular disease, disease prevention, hypertension, weight loss; External: aging skin, fungal infection	bulk, capsules, juice, tablets, tea, commercial skin care products	Hypotensive potential (see Chapter 17). Don't combine oral pomegranate with heart medications.
Psyllium (*Plantago ovata, P. psyllium*)	seed	Internal: constipation, diabetes, diarrhea, hyperglycemia, hyperlipidemia, weight loss; External: hair care	bulk, capsules, powder, tablets	Cholesterol-lowering potential (see Chapter 17). If you have diabetes, talk with your doctor before using. Don't use if you have problems swallowing or are prone to bowel obstruction. For topical treatments, soak the seeds in water to release the mucilage.
Pine bark: See Maritime pine				
Red clover (*Trifolium pratense*)	flower	acne, benign prostatic hypertrophy (BPH), breast pain (mastaglia), menopausal symptoms, osteoporosis	capsules, liquid extract, powder, tincture, tablets, tea	Anticoagulant/antiplatelet, estrogenic potential (see Chapter 17).

Name	Medicinal Parts	Key Uses	Available Forms	Safety Issues and Advice
Reishi (*Ganoderma lucidum*)	mushroom	altitude sickness, cancer, infectious disease, stress	bulk, capsules, liquid extract, powder, tea, tincture	Antiplatelet/anticoagulant, hypotensive, immunomodulating potential (see Chapter 17).
Rhodiola (*Rhodiola rosea*); also known as roseroot or golden root	root	depression, low energy, female infertility, immune support, stress	capsules, liquid extract, tablets, tea, tincture	Rhodiola has no known side effects or interactions.
Rice bran (*Oryza sativa*)	seed (outer hull)	Internal: hyperlipidemia, kidney support; External: atopic dermatitis	bulk, herbal oil, powder	Excessive doses can cause diarrhea and cramping. People prone to bowel obstructions shouldn't use it. Both rice bran and rice bran oil can lower cholesterol (defatted rice bran doesn't). Topically, rice bran can be used in a bath or applied directly (as a powder).
Rooibos (*Aspalathus linearis*)	leaf, stem	allergies, age-related cognitive decline, Alzheimer's disease and dementia, nausea and vomiting	bulk, liquid extract, powder, tea, tincture	Rooibos has no known side effects or interactions.
Rose (*Rosa canina, R. spp.*)	flower, hip (fruit)	Internal: disease prevention; External: aging skin, sun protection	capsules, tablets, tea, commercial skin care products, rose essential oil (*Rosa damascena*), rose hip seed oil, rose water	Rose hips (the fruit that grows after the flower has gone) contain high levels of ascorbic acid and are considered safe, although excessive doses can cause nausea and might interfere with nutrient absorption.
Rosemary (*Rosmarinus officinalis*)	leaf	Internal: acid indigestion (dyspepsia). indigestion and upset stomach; External: deodorant, hair loss, muscle and joint pain	bulk, capsules, powder, tea, tincture, essential oil, herbal oil, lotion	Don't take the essential oil internally.
Sage (*Salvia officinalis, S. lavandulaefolia*)	leaf	Internal: Alzheimer's disease and dementia, cognitive function and memory; External: cold sores, deodorant, viral infection	bulk, powder, tea, tincture, essential oil	Hypoglycemic, hypertensive, sedative potential; contains salicylates (see Chapter 17). Pregnant women should avoid sage. If you're buying essential oil, don't mistake it for clary sage (*Salvia sclarea*); don't use essential oil internally.
Saint John's wort (*Hypericum perforatum*)	flower, root	Internal: addictions and alcoholism, depression, menopausal symptoms, menstrual symptoms and PMS; External: bacterial infection, burns, ear infection, inflammatory skin disorders, minor wounds	bulk, capsules, liquid extract, powder, tablets, tea, tincture, herbal oil	Can cause insomnia, GI discomfort, and increased sun sensitivity. Don't take internally if you're pregnant or have any diagnosed psychiatric condition; because Saint John's wort can interfere with many drugs, talk with your doctor before using it. Store in the dark—its constituents are destroyed by light. Extracts are typically standardized to contain between 0.3 and 0.5 percent hypericin and/or 5 percent hyperforin.

Name	Medicinal Parts	Key Uses	Available Forms	Safety Issues and Advice
Sangre de grado (*Croton lechleri*)	bark, resin	Internal: diarrhea, foodborne illness (food poisoning); External: insect bites and stings, minor wounds, poisonous plants, viral infection	liquid extract	Sangre de grado has no known side effects or interactions.
Saw palmetto (*Serenoa repens*)	fruit	benign prostatic hyperplasia (BPH), cancer, hair loss	capsules, liquid extract, tablets, tincture	Anticoagulant/antiplatelet, antiestrogenic, sedative potential (see Chapter 17). If you're treating BPH, you'll need to wait at least a month or two before you see results. Standardized extracts contain between 80 and 95 percent fatty acids.
Schisandra (*Schisandra chinensis*)	fruit	cognitive function and memory, immune support, liver disease, male sexual dysfunction, stress	capsules, liquid extract, tablets, tincture	Schisandra can cause heartburn and other GI symptoms. Avoid if you have peptic ulcers or gastroesophageal reflux disease (GERD).
Slippery elm (*Ulmus rubra*)	inner bark	canker sores, cough and sore throat, oral pain	liquid extract, lozenges, powder, syrup	Can cause reactions in individuals sensitive to tree pollen. The traditional method for using slippery elm externally is to prepare a paste, or poultice, from the powdered inner bark. Commercial lozenges are probably a better option for sore throats.
Soy (*Glycine max*)	bean	diabetes, disease prevention, hair loss, hyperlipidemia, menopausal symptoms, osteoporosis, weight loss	bulk, capsules, powder	Estrogenic potential (see Chapter 17). Soy can cause minor GI symptoms (and is a fairly common food allergen). Avoid if you're taking a MAO inhibitor for depression.
Tea (*Camellia sinensis*)	leaf, stem	Internal: aging skin, allergies, asthma, bloating and water retention, diarrhea, disease prevention, inflammatory skin disorders, low energy, osteoporosis, sun protection, weight loss; External: dandruff, hair care, hair color, hair loss, oral care, sun protection, warts, viral infection	bulk, capsules, liquid extract, tea, tincture, commercial products (hair, skin/sun, oral care)	Stimulant (see Chapter 17). There are three types of tea, all the same species: green tea is unfermented, oolong is partially fermented, and black tea is completely fermented (green tea seems to have the highest levels of beneficial polyphenols).
Tea tree (*Melaleuca alternifolia*)	leaf	acne, athlete's foot, bacterial and fungal infection, burns, canker sores, cuts and scrapes, dandruff, deodorant, head lice, insect bites and stings, minor wounds, oily skin, oral care, oral pain, ringworm	commercial products (hair, skin, oral care), essential oil	Tea tree oil can cause skin reactions. Do not use internally—it's extremely toxic. To treat a vaginal infection, dilute essential oil and use as a douche. If you use tea tree oil to treat bad breath (diluted in water) or canker sores, be sure you don't swallow it.
Tinospora (*Tinospora cordifolia*)	stem	allergies	capsules, powder	Hypoglycemic, immunomodulating potential (see Chapter 17).
Tulsi (*Ocimum tenuiflorum, O. sanctum*); also known as holy basil	leaf, stem, seed	diabetes, immune support, infectious diseases, stress	capsules, powder	

Name	Medicinal Parts	Key Uses	Available Forms	Safety Issues and Advice
Turmeric (*Curcuma longa*)	rhizome	acid indigestion (dyspepsia), Alzheimer's disease and dementia, arthritis, cancer, hypertension, weight loss	capsules, liquid extract, powder, tablets, tincture	Anticoagulant/antiplatelet potential (see Chapter 17). Avoid if you have gallbladder problems.
Valerian (*Valeriana officinalis*)	rhizome, root	anxiety, insomnia	capsules, liquid extract, powder, tablets, tea, tincture	Sedative (see Chapter 17). Can cause headache, uneasiness, and even insomnia in some people. Avoid if you're taking antianxiety medications. Valerian tastes (and smells) terrible—many people prefer tablets or capsules over liquid remedies. It may take as long as three weeks of continuous use to obtain benefits.
Vitex (*Vitex agnus-castus*); also known as chasteberry	fruit, seed	Internal: breast pain (mastaglia), female infertility, menstrual symptoms and PMS; External: insect repellant	capsules, liquid extract, topical solution	Estrogenic potential (see Chapter 17). Don't combine with antidepressants or other psychotropic drugs.
Willow (*Salix alba*)	bark	Internal: back pain, headache; External: oily hair	capsules, liquid extract, tablet, tincture	Anticoagulant/antiplatelet potential; contains salicylates (see Chapter 17). Don't give to children or teenagers with viral infections, as it carries the same risk for Reye's syndrome that aspirin does.
Witch hazel (*Hamamelis virginiana*)	leaf, bark	allergies, bacterial infection, burns, cuts and scrapes, ear infection, hemorrhoids, insect bites and stings, minor wounds, oily hair and skin, poisonous plants	commercial products ("astringent" lotion, cream, gel), liquid extract	Don't take internally; don't apply to deep or open wounds. Can cause contact sensitivity.
Yarrow (*Achillea millefolium*)	aerial parts	deodorant, minor wounds, muscle and joint pain	liquid extract, tincture	Anticoagulant/antiplatelet potential; *Asteraceae/Compositae* family (see Chapter 17). If you're treating a cut, be sure to clean it first: yarrow will quickly stop blood flow and may trap bacteria in the wound.
Yohimbe (*Pausinystalia yohimbe*)	bark	female sexual dysfunction, male sexual dysfunction	capsules, liquid extract, powder, tablets, tincture	Hypertensive, hypotensive potential (see Chapter 17). Can cause insomnia, anxiety, headache, and nausea. Avoid if you have heart disease, BPH, diabetes, depression, high (or low) blood pressure, or kidney or liver disease.

Additional Resources

American Association of Naturopathic Physicians (AANP)

Provides information on naturopathy and a directory of licensed naturopathic doctors (NDs). *www.naturopathic.org*

American Association of Acupuncture and Oriental Medicine

Includes information on Traditional Chinese Medicine (TCM), plus a search function to help you find a licensed TCM practitioner in your area. *www.aaaomonline.org*

American Botanical Council (ABC)

A nonprofit research and educational foundation that provides information on individual herbs and news related to herbalism. *www.herbalgram.org*

American Chiropractic Association

Information on chiropractic and a search function to help you find a licensed chiropractor near you. *www.amerchiro.org*

American Herbalists Guild

The primary trade group of herbal practitioners in the United States. Offers a state-by-state search function to help you find an herbalist in your area. *www.americanherbalistsguild.com*

American Herbal Products Association (AHPA)

The trade association for manufacturers of herbal products, including dietary supplements. *www.ahpa.org*

The Alternative Medicine Foundation

A nonprofit group that provides information on herbal medicine and several complementary and alternative medicine (CAM) modalities that incorporate herbs. *www.amfoundation.org*

Balanced Healing Medical Center

Provides information about balancing the best of conventional medicine, alternative medicine, and research methods to facilitate healing. Offers herbs, supplements, and solutions for a variety of conditions. *www.balancedhealing.com*

Herb Research Foundation

A nonprofit group that provides information on research, legislation, and other developments related to herbs. *www.herbs.org*

National Association for Holistic Aromatherapy

Provides information on aromatherapy and a membership guide that can direct you to an aromatherapist in your area. *www.naha.org*

National Center for Complementary and Alternative Medicine (NCCAM)

The official site of NCCAM, the government agency in charge of scientific research on complementary and alternative medicine (CAM). *www.nccam.nih.gov*

Office of Dietary Supplements (ODS)

This is the government agency in charge of all dietary supplements, including herbal products. *www.ods.od.nih.gov*

Organic Consumers Association

A nonprofit group that encourages sustainable organic farming; search for information on a particular herb or get a list of retailers that sell organic products near you. www.*organicconsumers.org*

PubMed Central

PubMed Central is a free archive of biomedical and life sciences journal articles. *www.ncbi.nlm.nih.gov*

INDEX